MW01233950

Keto Diet for Women Over 50

& Keto Chaffle Recipes

The ultimate ketogenic guide for burn fat quickly, live a healthy lifestyle after 50 and meal plan with a lot of low-carb recipes for beginners

By

Serena Green

Table of contents

KETO CHAFFLE RECIPES 2020

KETO DIET FOR WOMEN OVER 50

Regain Body Confidence Through Diabetes Prevention, Weight Loss Exercises, Hormones Balancing and Anti-Aging Solutions [Keto Chaffle Recipes] 2020 Ketogenic Guide

BY: Serena Green

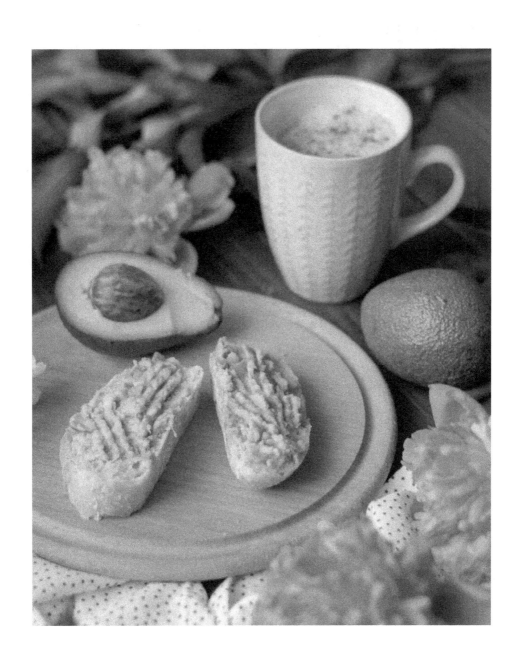

PART ONE

Introduction to Ketogenic Diet

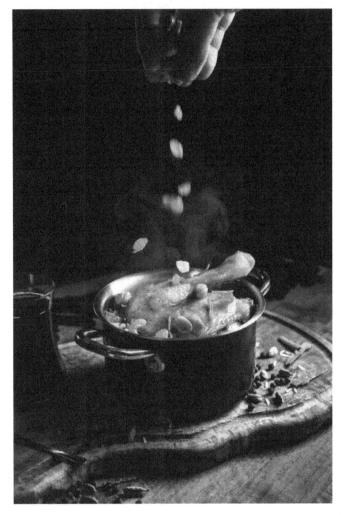

The keto diet is a low-carb and high-fat diet. It brings down glucose and insulin levels and moves the body's digestion away from carbs and towards fat and ketones.

"Ketogenic" is a term used for a low-carb diet. The thought is for you to get more calories from protein and fat and less from sugars.

The ketogenic diet is a high-fat, satisfactory protein, low-sugar diet that in medication is utilized essentially to get troublesome control (unmanageable) epilepsy in youngsters. The diet forces the body to consume fats rather than starches. Typically, the starches contained in nourishment are changed over into glucose, which is then shipped around the body and is especially significant in filling mind work.

Ketogenic diets can cause huge decreases in glucose and insulin levels. This, alongside the expanded ketones, has various health benefits.

How Food Affects Your Body

The nourishment we eat gives our bodies the "information" and materials they have to work appropriately. In the event that we don't get the correct information, our metabolic procedures endure, and our health decreases.

In the event that women get an excessive amount of nourishment or nourishment that gives their body an inappropriate guidelines, we can get overweight, undernourished, and in danger for the advancement of sicknesses and conditions, for example, joint inflammation, diabetes, and coronary illness.

The supplements in nourishment enables the cells in our bodies to perform their fundamental capacities. This statement from a well-known coursebook depicts how the supplements in nourishment are fundamental for our physical working.

"Supplements are the feeding substances in nourishment that are fundamental for the development, advancement, and support for the body capacities. Fundamental stated that if a supplement is absent, parts of capacity, and therefore, human health decrease. At the point when supplement consumption doesn't normally meet the supplement needs directed by the cell action, the metabolic procedures delayed down or even stopped."

To put it plainly, what we eat is fundamental to our health.

The keto diet requires sticking to a very low-carb, high-fat diet so as to place your body into a metabolic state called ketosis. This makes your body increasingly productive at consuming fat.

The ketogenic diet can bring about a drop in the drive when beginning the diet, as the dieter will encounter side effects of carb withdrawal and conceivably the keto influenza.

When the withdrawal and influenza-like side effects have passed, and the dieter has adjusted to the lower-carb way of life, the charisma will in all probability reset and conceivably be superior to earlier because of weight loss from the diet.

While the drive cautioning got a great deal of reputation in the media,

In other words, supplements give our bodies directions about how to work. In this sense, nourishment can be viewed as a wellspring of "information" for the body.

Pondering nourishment along these lines gives us a perspective on the sustenance that goes past calories or grams, great food sources, or awful food sources. This view drivesus to concentrate on nourishments we ought to incorporate rather than food sources to avoid.

Rather than review nourishment as the adversary, we look to nourishment as an approach to make health and diminish malady by helping the body look after capacity.

Kidney and heart harm

Since the body is low on electrolytes and liquid over the expanded pee, that can prompt a loss of electrolytes, for example, sodium, magnesium, and potassium. This can make individuals inclined to intense kidney damage.

Drying out is not kidding and may bring about lightheadedness, kidney damage, or kidney stones.

This may place the dieter in danger of cardiovascular arrhythmia, as electrolytes are fundamental for the typical thumping of the heart.

"Electrolyte lacks are not kidding and may bring about a sporadic heartbeat, which can be destructive,"

Yo-yo dieting designs

The keto diet can likewise prompt yo-yo dieting since individuals experience issues remaining on the prohibitive diet forever.

That can have other negative impacts on the body.

Other effects

Other reactions can incorporate awful breath, weakness, obstruction, sporadic menstrual cycles, diminished bone thickness, and rest issues.

Then there are other impacts that are not very much considered, for the most part, since it's difficult to follow dieters on a long haul premise to discover the enduring impacts of the eating plan.

Wholesome concerns

"There is a dread among health specialists that such high admissions of unhealthful fats would have a long haul negative impact," she clarified. Weight loss can often befuddle the information for the time being. This is on the grounds that when overweight individuals get in shape, paying little heed to how they do it, they often end up with better blood lipids and blood glucose levels.

The keto diet is additionally incredibly low in specific natural products, vegetables, grains, and vegetables that are by and the large idea of as healthy. Without these nourishments, individuals on a diet can pass up fiber, certain nutrients, minerals, and phytochemicals that lone come in these nourishments. That has critical human health impacts over the long haul, for example, bone loss and expanded danger of interminable sicknesses.

Sodium

The mix of fat, sugar, and bunches of sodium (salt) can make cheap food more delectable to certain individuals. Yet, diets high in sodium can prompt water maintenance, which is the reason you may feel puffy, enlarged, or swollen in the wake of eating inexpensive food.

A diet high in sodium is likewise hazardous for individuals with pulse conditions. Sodium can hoist circulatory strain and put weight on your heart and cardiovascular framework.

As indicated by one examination, around 90 percent of grown-ups belittle how much sodium is in their cheap food meals.

The examination overviewed 993 grown-ups and found that their speculations were multiple times lower than the real number (1,292 milligrams). This implies sodium gauges were off by in excess of 1,000 mg.

Remember that the AHA prescribes grown-ups eat close to 2,300 milligrams of sodium for each day. One cheap food dinner could have a large portion of your day's worth.

Impact on the respiratory framework

Overabundance calories from inexpensive food meals can cause weight gain. This may lead to weight.

Corpulence builds your hazard for respiratory issues, including asthma and brevity of breath.

The additional pounds can place pressure on your heart and lungs, and side effects may appear even with little effort. You may see trouble breathing when you're strolling, climbing stairs, or working out.

For youngsters, the danger of respiratory issues is particularly clear. One investigation found that youngsters who eat inexpensive food at any rate three times each week are bound to create asthma.

Impact on the focal sensory system

Inexpensive food may fulfill the hunger for the time being, yet long haul results are more negative.

Individuals who ate cheap food and prepared baked goods are 51 percent bound to create sadness than individuals who don't eat those nourishments or eat not many of them.

Impact on the conceptive framework

The fixings in lousy nourishment and cheap food may affect your richness.

One examination found that prepared nourishment contains phthalates. Phthalates are synthetic substances that can interfere with how hormones act in your body. Introduction to significant levels of these synthetics could prompt regenerative issues, including birth absconds.

Impact on the integumentary framework (skin, hair, nails)

The nourishments you eat may affect your skin's appearance, yet it probably won't be the nourishments you think.

Previously, chocolate and oily nourishments like pizza have assumed the fault for skin break out breakouts. However, as per the Mayo Clinic, it's starches. Carb-rich nourishments lead to glucose spikes, and these abrupt hops in glucose levels may trigger skin inflammation. Find nourishments that help battle skin break out.

Youngsters and youths who eat cheap food at any rate three times each week are additionally bound to create skin inflammation, as indicated by one investigation. Dermatitis is a skin condition that causes aggravated patches of excited, bothersome skin.

Impact on the skeletal framework (bones)

Carbs and sugar in cheap food and handled nourishment can expand acids in your mouth. These acids can separate tooth lacquer. As tooth veneer vanishes, microorganisms can grab hold, and depressions may create.

Weight can likewise prompt inconveniences with bone thickness and bulk. Individuals who are hefty have a more serious hazard for falling and breaking bones. It's critical to continue practicing to construct muscles, which bolster your bones and keep up a healthy diet to limit bone loss.

Regardless of efforts to bring issues to light and make women more intelligent customers, one investigation found that the measure of calories, fat, and sodium in inexpensive food meals remains, to a great extent, unaltered.

As women get busier and eat out more oftentimes, it could have antagonistic impacts for the individual and America's healthcare framework.

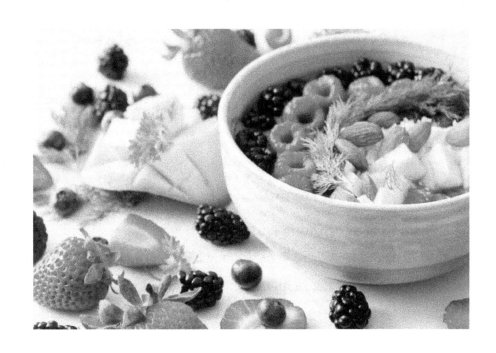

Why Do the Ketogenic Diet

KETOGENIC works by exhausting your body of its store of sugar, so it will begin to separate protein and fat for vitality, causing ketosis (and weight loss).

1. Helps in weight loss

It takes more work to transform fat into vitality than it takes to transform carbs into vitality. Along these lines, a ketogenic diet can assist speed with increasing weight loss. Furthermore, since the diet is high in protein, it doesn't leave you hungry as other diets do. In a meta-examination of 13 diverse randomized controlled preliminaries, five results uncovered huge weight loss from a ketogenic diet.

2. Diminishes skin break out

There are various reasons for skin break out, and one might be identified with diet and glucose. Eating a diet balancedprepared and refined starches can modify gut microscopic organisms and affects increasingly sensational glucose variances, the two of which can have an impact on skin health. Therefore, by diminishing carb admission, it is anything but an unexpected that a ketogenic diet could decrease a few instances of skin inflammation.

3. May help diminish the danger of malignancy

The ketogenic diet has been tested a lot for how it might help forestall or even treat certain malignant growths. One investigation found that the ketogenic diet might be an appropriate corresponding treatment to chemotherapy and radiation in individuals with malignancy. This is because of the way that it would cause more oxidative worry in malignancy cells than in ordinary cells.

Other theories recommend that in light of the fact that the ketogenic diet decreases high glucose, it could diminish insulin entanglements, which might be related to certain tumors.

4. Improves heart health

When the ketogenic diet is accessed in a healthy way (which looks at avocados as a healthy fat rather than pork skins), there is some proof that the diet can improve heart health by lessening cholesterol. One examination found that HDL ("great") cholesterol levels fundamentally expanded in those following the keto diet. The LDL ("terrible") cholesterol went down essentially.

5. May secure mind working

More research is required into the keto diet and the mind. A few investigations propose that the keto diet offers neuroprotective benefits. These may help treat or forestall conditions as Alzheimer Parkinson's, and even some rest issue. One investigation even found that youngsters following a ketogenic diet had improved sharpness and psychological working.

6. *Possibly lessens seizures*

It's the idea that the blend of fat, protein, and carbs modifies the manner in which the body utilizes vitality, bringing about ketosis. Ketosis is a raised degree of ketone bodies in the blood.

Ketosis can prompt a decrease in seizures in individuals with epilepsy.

7. *Improves health in women with PCOS*

Polycystic ovarian disorder (PCOS) is an endocrine issue that causes augmented ovaries with pimples. A high-sugar diet can contrarily influence those with PCOS.

There aren't numerous clinical examinations on the ketogenic diet and PCOS. One pilot study that included five women over a 24-week time frame found that the ketogenic diet:

- increased weight loss
- aided hormone balance
- improved luteinizing hormone (LH)/follicle-invigorating hormone (FSH) proportions
- improved fasting insulin

Keto is often recommended for kids who experience the ill effects of the specific issue (like Lennox-Gastaut disorder or Rett disorder) and don't react to seizure prescription, as indicated by the Epilepsy Foundation.

(1) They note that keto can diminish the number of seizures these kids have considerably, with 10 to 15 percent turning out to be sans seizure. In other

cases, it might likewise assist patients with diminishing the portion of their drug.

The keto diet may likewise be advantageous for grown-ups with epilepsy.

Be that as it may, the ketogenic diet likewise has a lot of strong research backing up its benefits. Truth be told, it has been seen as superior to most diets at assisting individuals with:

- Epilepsy
- Type 2 Diabetes
- Type 1 Diabetes
- High Blood Pressure
- Alzheimer's infection
- Parkinson's infection
- Chronic Inflammation
- High Blood Sugar Levels
- Obesity
- Heart Disease
- Polycystic Ovary Syndrome
- Fatty Liver Disease
- Cancer
- Migraines

Regardless of whether you are not in danger from any of these conditions, the ketogenic diet can be useful for you as well. A portion of the benefits that the vast majority experience are:

- Better cerebrum work

- A decline in aggravation

- An increment in vitality

- Improved body arrangement

As should be obvious, the ketogenic diet has a wide cluster of benefits, yet is it any superior to other diets?

8. Treating Epilepsy — The Origins of The Ketogenic Diet

The excellent primary examination on epilepsy and the ketogenic diet wasn't distributed until some other time, in 1998

Of around 150 kids, and almost every one of them had multiple seizures every week regardless of taking in any event two seizure-decreasing meds.

The kids were given a ketogenic diet for a one-year preliminary.

Following three months, about 34% of the kids, or marginally more than 33%, had over a 90% abatement in seizures.

It was expressed that the ketogenic diet is "more viable than a considerable lot of the new anticonvulsant prescriptions and is very much endured by kids and families when it is successful." Not just was the ketogenic diet supportive. However, it was more useful than some ordinarily utilized medications.

9. Improving Blood Pressure With the Ketogenic Diet

A low-sugar diet is more successful than a low-fat and moderate-fat diet at decreasing pulse. Constraining starches even creates preferable outcomes over the blend of a low-fat diet and a weight-loss/pulse tranquilize.

10. The Power to Improve Alzheimer's Disease

Alzheimer's malady patients concur with organic chemistry as well." high sugar admission intensifies intellectual performance and conduct in patients with Alzheimer's infection." This implies eating more starches mess more up in the cerebrum. Will the inverse (eating fewer carbs) improve cerebrum work?

Other benefits that ketone bodies have on mental health care:

- They forestall neuronal loss.
- They save neuron work.
- They ensure synapses against various sorts of damage.

The Benefits of Following Ketogenic Diet

Picking a ketogenic diet for diabetes, the board offers a scope of significant benefits.

Being in a condition of healthful ketosis outstandingly prompts huge improvement in blood glucose control and weight loss.

Other regular benefits gave include:

- Reduced reliance on taking drugs
- Improvements in insulin affectability
- Lower circulatory strain
- Usually enhancements in cholesterol levels.

In this guide, we survey the science behind the ketogenic diet and how it attempts to give these various benefits.

Weight loss and support

An essential advantage of the ketogenic diet is its capacity to accomplish fast weight loss Restricting starches enough to be in a condition of ketosis prompts both a noteworthy which reduce in muscle versus fats and increasing and maintenance of the bulk.

Studies had show that low-carb, ketogenic diets can accomplish solid weight loss over an all-inclusive period. A large individuals had the option to lose, by and large, 15 kg over a time of a year. This was 3 kg that is more than the low-fat diet utilized in the investigation accomplished.

Blood glucose control

The other primary explanation behind individuals with diabetes to follow a ketogenic diet is its capacity to lower and balance out glucose levels.

Starch is the supplement (macronutrient) that raises glucose the most. Since ketogenic diets are low in starch, they dispense with the bigger ascents in glucose.

Ketogenic diets demonstrate them to be successful at diminishing HbA1c – a long haul proportion of blood glucose control. A normal decrease in HbA1c levels of 17 mmol/mol (1.5%) for individuals with type 2 diabetes.

Individuals with other sorts of diabetes, for example, type 1 diabetes and LADA, ought to likewise hope to see a solid decrease in glucose levels and an improvement in charge.

Note that if an improvement in blood glucose control is kept up over various years, this can lessen the danger of intricacies happening.

It is significant that anybody on insulin, or otherwise in danger of hypos, plays it safe to forestall hypos happening. Address your PCP for help with this

Diminishing dependency on diabetes prescription

Since they're so successful at lessening glucose levels, ketogenic diets have the extra advantage of helping individuals with type 2 diabetes to diminish their reliance on diabetes medicine.

Individuals on insulin and other hypo-causing prescription (for example, sulphonylureas and glinides) may need to lessen their portions ahead of time of beginning a ketogenic diet to forestall hypos. consult your primary care physician for guidance on this.

Insulin affectability

A ketogenic diet has been appeared to help re-establish insulin affectability, as it dispenses with the underlying driver of insulin obstruction – which is too significant levels of insulin in the body.

This diet advances supported times of low insulin, as low degrees of starch means lower levels of insulin.

A high starch diet resembles placing petroleum on the fire of insulin obstruction. High sugar implies a more prominent requirement for insulin, and this aggravates insulin opposition.

By correlation, a ketogenic diet, turns insulin levels down, as fat is the macronutrient that requires the least insulin.

Getting the degrees of insulin down additionally assists with fat consumption, in light of the fact that high insulin levels forestall the breakdown of fat. At the point when insulin levels drop for various hours, the body can separate fat cells.

Hypertension control

It is assessed that 16 million individuals are living with a hypertension in the UK.

Scope of health conditions are related to hypertension, for example, coronary illness, stroke, and kidney malady. It is likewise a component of metabolic inbalance

Various examinations have showed that a ketogenic diet can diminish circulatory strain levels in individuals that are overweight or with type 2 diabetes.

Cholesterol levels

Ketogenic diets, for the most part, bring about enhancements of cholesterol levels. It is common for LDL cholesterol levels to go down, and HDL cholesterol levels go up, which is healthy.

Perhaps the most grounded proportion of healthy cholesterol is the proportion of absolute cholesterol to HDL. This can be effectively found by taking your complete cholesterol result and partitioning it by your HDL result.

On the off chance that the number you get is 3.5 or lower, this demonstrates healthy cholesterol. The research examines show that ketogenic diets are generally viable at improving this proportion of cholesterol health.

Note that a few people may show an expansion in LDL and all-out cholesterol subsequent to beginning a ketogenic. This is normally viewed as a negative sign, yet in the event that your absolute cholesterol to HDL proportion is acceptable, this doesn't really speak to compounding in heart health.

Cholesterol is a confusing subject, and your PCP is the best wellspring of exhortation if your cholesterol levels change essentially on a ketogenic diet.

More grounded mental performance

Mental clearness, an expanded capacity to center, and a superior memory are other ordinarily announced benefits of eating a ketogenic diet.

Expanding admission of healthy fats with omega-3, for example, those found in slick fish like salmon, fish, and mackerel, can improve the state of mind and learning capacity. This is on the grounds that omega-3 expands an unsaturated fat called DHA that makes up between 15 to 30 percent of the women cerebrum

The creation of beta-hydroxybutyrate, a form of ketone, enables backing to long haul memory work.

Satiety

Ketogenic diets effects affect hunger. When the body adjusts to being in a condition of ketosis, it becomes acclimated to getting vitality from separating muscle to fat ratio, and this can lessen hunger and desires.

They are viable at:

- Reducing desires
- Helping you feel full for more
- Reducing inclination for sugary nourishments

Weight loss because of a ketogenic diet can help lower leptin levels, which can improve leptin affectability and advantage satiety accordingly.

Candida

Ketogenic diets can be acceptable at lessening thrush and yeast contaminations as they lower glucose, which diminishes glucose being dropped in the pee.

It is glucose in the pee that microbes feed off that prompts a prolific rearing places for the yeast and bacterial diseases.

A higher admission of a soaked unsaturated fat called lauric corrosive – found in coconut oil, a staple keto nourishment – has been appeared to have hostile to microbial properties. It can murder off candida albican and help with yeast contaminations.

Improving vitality levels and rest

Each day 4 or 5 on a ketogenic diet, a great many people report an expansion as a rule vitality levels and an absence of longings for carbs. The instrument here includes both an adjustment of insulin levels and promptly accessible wellspring of vitality for our cerebrum and body tissues.

Rest upgrades are more of a secret. Studies have demonstrated that ketogenic dieting improves rest by diminishing REM and expanding moderate wave rest designs. While the definite instrument is misty, it likely is identified with the complex biochemical movements, including the cerebrum's utilization of ketones for vitality joined with other body tissues straightforwardly consuming fat.

Helping gastrointestinal and gallbladder health (less indigestion and heartburn, less hazard for gallstones, improved processing, less gas, and swelling)

It is notable that grain-based nourishments, nightshade vegetables like potatoes and tomatoes, and sugary nourishments improve the probability of indigestion and acid reflux. Therefore, it's not astounding that eating a low-carb diet improves these indications and really goes up against the root issues of irritation, bacterial issues, and immune system reactions.

Identified with this, it is realized that adjustments in diet quickly and reproducibly changes the human gut microbiome. A large group of issues is fundamentally diminished or expelled because of microbiome changes on a ketogenic diet.

By removing the starch in the nourishment, It can essentially fix each gastrointestinal issue that influences individuals today.

Research additionally shows that carbs in the diet are one of the key elements for gallstones. To some degree, irrationally, eating an adequate measure of fat when carb admission is down assisting clear with excursion the gallbladder and keep things running easily to keep gallstones from forming.

Helping the eyes (progressively stable vision; less hazard for waterfalls)

As any diabetic will let you know, it is notable that high glucose detrimentally affects visual perception and prompts an expanded hazard for waterfalls. It's therefore not astounding that keeping glucose levels low improves eye and vision health, as a gazillion people have shared on the web, and as related diabetes inquires about has demonstrated.

Picking up muscle and improving continuance

BHB, explicitly, has been appeared to advance muscle gain. Joined with huge amounts of narrative proof throughout the years, there is a whole development behind jocks utilizing a ketogenic way to deal with acquiring muscle and less fat (commonly muscle gain likewise accompanies fat addition, so there's justifiable consideration being given toward forestalling this).

Checking diabetes, corpulence, and metabolic disorder while saving muscle loss

Ketogenic dieting is incredibly viable for some individuals with both sort I and types II diabetes for every one of the reasons examined above identified with keeping glucose levels and insulin under tight restraints.

Scientific Proof That the Ketogenic Diet Is Helpful

The low-starch, high-fat ketogenic, or "keto," diet, researchers are attempting to examine it – from how it impacts irritation in mind to its consequences for weight and heart health, just as some other potential health dangers.

The ketogenic diet attempts to bring sugars down to under 5 percent of an individual's day by day caloric admission – which means dispensing with most grains, natural products, bland vegetables, vegetables, and desserts. Rather, it replaces those calories with fat. That fat is transformed into ketone bodies, which are an elective vitality source: other than glucose got from starches, ketones from fat are the main fuel the mind can utilize.

What We Know

The effects of ketogenic diets on aggravation in mind, got inquisitive about the ketogenic diet when attempting to treat the irritation that endures for days after an individual endures a stroke. At the point when he took a stab at actuating a ketogenic state in mice with stroke wounds. Blocking glucose digestion attempted to stifle fiery qualities, which thusly helped stroke mending.

The mitigating impact of ketosis on stroke recuperation is likely a similar impact that helps kids with particular sorts of seizures, Ketogenic diets have been utilized as a treatment for certain forms of epilepsy for just about a century.

It's unimaginably incredible for the keto diet. Curtailing starches, there are such a large number of metabolic benefits. The body forms the rest of the starches all the more effectively. Thus it requires substantially less insulin.

Performing more preliminaries focused on individuals with type 2 diabetes. In the controlled preliminaries, a ketogenic state has demonstrated a guarantee in improving human glucose control and diminishing the requirement for diabetes prescriptions.

What We Don't Know

One major obstacle to the information about the keto diet's effect on people is that a considerable lot of the benefits – lessening irritation in the cerebrum, improving results after mind damage, and expanding life expectancy – have just been found in examines in mice.

Far less clinical investigations have been done in people outside of seizure counteraction since ketosis is a troublesome state to keep up, maintaining a strategic distance from carbs, including natural products, bread, vegetables, and the incidental office birthday cake isn't possible for some individuals over the long haul.

Without peer-inspected clinical preliminaries, a large number of the benefits stay narrative. For example, Weiss himself has been on a low-carb high-fat (however not carefully ketogenic) diet for over a half year, and cases he improves. However, he's unmistakable about what he knows and what he doesn't. He's shed pounds, and his marginal pre-diabetes is no more.

However, that may be on the grounds that he's eating less prepared nourishment, resting better, or getting a charge out of praises on his new build.

With regards to the most colorful cases from health and diet masters –, for example, keto diets bringing about happiness, subjective lifts, and enhancements in anything from kidney capacity to malignant growth treatment – "We simply don't have the information on that yet.

The scientists concur that the diet itself isn't characteristically perilous. If you have any ailment, in the event that you take any medication whatsoever – there are bunches of things that change how drugs work in our bodies, and nourishment is unquestionably one of them. In case you're rolling out a genuine improvement in your nourishment, you should converse with your primary care physician."

The web is buzzing with stories recounting the astonishing benefits of a ketogenic (or "keto") diet. The same old thing there, then, as consistently is set apart by the ascent and fall of another diet prevailing fashion – most enhanced by the web-based life reverberation chamber however, with little to recognize them.

This time, however, grabbed my eye. Not in a way that I am an unassumingly overweight multi-year old whose adoration for nourishment and drink is marginally more grounded than my longing to be skinny, and subsequently somebody who has been on a diet each January for in any event 20 years and now knows he needs he wonders. But since of the science behind it.

For a beginning, I initially started finding out about ketogenic diets on account of Ethan Weiss, whose scientific astuteness I regard. On the off chance that he has faith in the benefits of ketosis, then I should look somewhat nearer. Following 20 years of January diets, my very own experience recommended that nothing had any effect: you possibly shed pounds in the event that you took in fewer calories than you utilized, and on the off chance that you took in fewer calories than you utilized, then you were eager. Basic as that. Might it be able to be that a ketogenic diet truly was unique?

Today In: Innovation

All things considered, the standard bodes well. Peculiarly named "ketone bodies" are really atoms that go about as the body's natural back-up fuel supply when glucose is rare. Ordinarily, we just enter ketosis (where ketone bodies gather in the blood) when we starve ourselves – medium-term or by missing a feast, however, for a few days at a time. Our digestion then changes to fat-consuming and changes over put away fat particles into ketone bodies that can control our muscles and mind in light of the fact that the glucose has run out. Being in ketosis, then, sounds like an extraordinary method to consume off the fat. Then again, not eating for days doesn't sound a lot of fun.

It turns out you don't have to starve yourself to get into ketosis. You should simply expel sugar from the diet (not simply refined carbs, for example, sucrose or high fructose corn syrup, yet all carbs, including complex carbs and starches as well). When the body has no wellspring of glucose, it needs to change to ketosis in light of the fact that the cerebrum needs either glucose or ketone bodies to endure. So regardless of how much protein or fat you eat, the body still needs to separate fat to ketone bodies to prop you up.

Advanced

A ketogenic diet, then, is any diet that changes your digestion to ketosis. What's more, the ones doing the rounds right now aren't the first or the main diets to do that. It is a very long while since the Atkins Diet rose to noticeable quality – and I saw direct the weight loss a few companions accomplished on Atkins. The Atkins diet is a ketogenic diet since it expels carbs from the diet and replaces them with protein. The astounding discovering was that Atkins devotees found they were significantly less eager than they expected, proposing that calories from protein caused you to feel increasingly fulfilled for more. They are feeling more full means readily eating less, and at last great weight loss.

In dieting, however, there is nothing of the sort as a free lunch (or so I thought). Adherence to the Atkins diet has reactions, and most stress is the effect on nitrogen balance from taking in so much protein. There is an undeniable danger of lack of hydration, and over the more extended term, kidney stones from the need to discharge such a lot of abundance nitrogen as urea.

So shouldn't something be said about the 21st-century adaptation? Keto today replaces the carbs with fats rather than protein. A run of the mill Atkins routine had 75% of calories from protein, 25% from fat, and <5% from carbs. On the other hand, the present keto diets advocate 75% of calories from fat, 25% from protein, and <5% from carbs. As protein admission isn't transformed from a run of the mill "adjusted" diet, any symptoms from nitrogen unevenness are flawlessly avoided.

In any case, shouldn't something be said about such fat? Definitely, that is found a good pace? All things considered, no. Most enlightening are the lipid profiles of Antarctic voyagers who have crossed the landmass by walking, hauling their own nourishment on sleds. That is just conceivable with nourishment that has the most elevated conceivable calorie to weight proportion – which means eating basically only spread. Furthermore, after months on an all-spread diet, the degree of LDL-cholesterol (often called "awful cholesterol") really decreases fundamentally. That isn't as astonishing as it sounds – while in ketosis, fats are being moved from stores towards the liver (where the ketone bodies are made), and that is the activity of HDL-cholesterol. LDL-cholesterol ordinarily moves abundance fat from the liver to the stores in the remainder of the body (henceforth the other way). So in ketosis, you would expect a lipid profile regularly thought to be healthier (higher HDL and lower LDL) regardless of how much fat was being expended.

In any case, if the benefits of Atkins on weight originated from the decreased yearning because of the continuing properties of the protein, then you shouldn't get that except if you beef up the protein segment of the diet. For reasons unknown, however, that the diminished craving results from the condition of ketosis itself. How you accomplish it doesn't generally make a difference.

So the science piles up – theoretically, in any event, I was unable to discover an imperfection in the cutting edge ketogenic diet. So I checked out it instead of my standard thing "low-everything" calorie confined January diet.

 Utilizing pee dipsticks, my ketone body level was continued above 6 moles/liter, proportionate to a "profound" ketosis.

Also, there it has remained for a month, while I appreciated the enjoyments of burgers bested with brie, kind sized prawn plates of mixed greens with avocado and sharp cream dressings and rich pork stroganoff with zucchini strips: three fat-loaded meals each and every day.

First, the benefits: when ketosis was entrenched three days in, I discovered I was rarely ravenous. I had no craving at all to nibble between meals (generally a major shortcoming), and bit by bit over a month, I wound up pondering nourishment – to the point missing lunch altogether was something that could happen "coincidentally."

I likewise found my fixation and concentration significantly improving. I had never had such a lot of vitality, and efficiency experienced the roof.

Running on the back-up batteries (the ketone bodies) is such a great amount of superior to fuelling yourself with carbs. For what reason was that? Simply on the grounds that the levels never decay (in any event for a plump individual like me, with an unlimited inventory of interior fat stores to consume). Paradoxically, when you eat carbs, the abundance is promptly saved as fat (for a blustery day) with the goal that blood glucose levels fall a couple of hours subsequent to eating, and that triggers the desire to eat once more, yet in addition a sentiment of declining vitality and fixation (that "late evening plunge" us 'carnivores' perceive very well indeed).

Furthermore, eating less did to be sure to convert into amazing weight loss (14lbs gone in less than a month), generally from the unattractive and unhealthy stomach fat stores, so my waistline contracted two scores on my belt as well. That is about twice as much weight-loss as my typical hopeless January diet can accomplish by making me continually ravenous.

There were even some unforeseen benefits I took note of. For instance, the measure of plaque on my teeth diminished to the right around zero (apparently in light of the fact that the plaque microscopic organisms need the dietary carbs to nourish off).

Shouldn't something be said about the drawbacks? Beside irritating my companions with steady stories of the benefits of a ketogenic diet (the recently changed over are consistently the noisiest evangelists), there were just two drawbacks I could consider.

The first is basically reasonable. Keeping carbs underneath 5% of absolute calories is a test. You need to check the sugar substance of everything that you eat, and you find tricky carbs stowing away in nearly everything pre-arranged. Eating out at eateries turns into a test, and as a visitor with loved ones practically inconceivable (except if they are additionally on a ketogenic diet or are unimaginably pleasing). Subsequently, arranging and planning nourishment turns into a fundamentally more noteworthy interest in your time and assets than it was before.

On similar lines, you do need to apply exact segment control as well – as the meals, high in fat, have a fatty thickness, you can accidentally eat such a large number of calories. What's more, even the keto diet can't violate the physical laws of the universe, for example, the protection of vitality – to shed pounds; you need to eat fewer calories than you need. It just methods you feel incredible while doing it.

The subsequent drawback was less difficult to stay away from. It is difficult to get enough fiber while following a ketogenic diet, primarily in light of the fact that most natural fiber sources additionally contain an excess of accessible starch (fiber is ordinarily an insoluble or unpalatable sugar polymer, so it's obvious it naturally coincides with absorbable carbs). The arrangement is basic: take a fiber supplement some women need 7 or 8 grams per day – from the principal day, you change to a ketogenic diet.

Toward the finish of my examination, I chose to watch the effect of eating some starch after very nearly a month being basically without a carb. Only

50g of carbs in one sitting (identical to a little prepared potato) quickly slaughtered ketosis. Inside 3 hours, urinary ketone body levels had tumbled to basically imperceptible – hunger returned, and the "psychological mist" began to dive.

Obviously, it then took very nearly 72 hours to restore "profound" ketosis after only one (for my situation conscious) snapshot of shortcoming. Three days of feeling piece garbage, ailing in vitality, since women denied their body its typical glucose fuel and the back-up batteries, the ketone bodies, were yet to cut in. Accomplishment on a ketogenic diet, therefore, unmistakably requires the sort of control commonly connected with a Zen ace.

This investigation outlines pleasantly the issue of an "adjusted" diet foundations for the digestion of an advanced human. Ketosis is delayed to set up yet exceptionally brisk to kill – a marvel researchers call hysteresis. What's more, there are generally excellent transformative purposes behind this set up: while a decent fuel, glucose, and other starches can harm the proteins that make up your cells and tissues.If glucose levels are permitted to get excessively high, the harm might be hopeless (as can occur in diabetes). To maintain a strategic distance from that, at any rate in healthy individuals, the body makes insulin when blood glucose levels begin to rise – and insulin tops the degree of glucose in the blood by training the liver to change over the overabundance into fat. Simultaneously, nonetheless, that insulin turns of ketosis (which is the reason ketosis finished so rapidly after I ate a prepared potato). That guarantees you are not setting down fat and consuming fat simultaneously (which would be an exceptionally wasteful utilization of nourishment assets).

In ancient times, development tuned our digestion, so we didn't promptly begin taking care of to our fat stores the minute nourishment became alarmed. People who did that would find that when a conceivably calamitous nourishment deficiency happened, they would have less fat put away as to be the first to capitulate. Obviously, today, when for a great many people in created nations, accessibility of calories is boundless, this hysteresis that once made us proficient currently makes us fat. Each ounce of abundance starch is put away as fat. However, those stores are not re-got to when your glucose is exhausted. Rather you are left inclination eager and ailing in vitality for some time – and with cheap food fries inside simple arrive at it's simply excessively enticing to refuel with carbs once more.

Ketosis was, some time ago, key to giving people an endurance advantage. The science, and my own understanding, proposes it can surely do likewise for people today. On the off chance that you haven't attempted it yet, perhaps you should.

PART 2

Health Concern for Women Over 50+ Menopause And Skin Sagging

Healthy maturing includes great propensities like eating healthy, evading regular prescription missteps, overseeing health conditions, getting suggested screenings, and being dynamic.

Getting more seasoned includes change, both negative and positive, yet you can appreciate maturing on the off chance that you comprehend what's new with your body and find a way to keep up your health.

A wide range of things happens to your body as you age. Your skin, bones, and even cerebrum may begin to carry on in an unexpected way. Try not to let the progressions that accompany mature age get you off guard.

Here is a portion of the normal ones:

- Your bones. Bones can become more slender and progressively weak in mature age, particularly in women, once in a while bringing about the delicate bone condition called osteoporosis. Diminishing bones and diminishing bone mass can place you in danger for falls that can happen without much of a stretch outcome in broken bones. Make certain to converse with your doctor about what you can do to forestall osteoporosis and falls.

- Your heart. While a healthy diet and standard exercise can keep your heart healthy, it might turn out to be somewhat amplified, your pulse may lower, and the dividers of the heart may thicken.

- Your mind and sensory system. In getting more seasoned can cause changes in your reflexes and even your faculties. While dementia is definitely not an ordinary outcome of mature age, it is basic for individuals to encounter some slight forgetfulness as they get more stated. Cells in the cerebrum and nerves can be harmed by the formation of plaques and tangles, irregularities that could, in the end, lead to dementia.

- Your stomach related framework. As you age, your stomach related tract turns out to be all the more firm and inflexible, and doesn't contract as often. This change can prompt issues, for example, obstruction, stomach torment, and sentiments of queasiness; a superior diet can help.

- Your faculties. You may see that your vision and hearing aren't exactly as sharp as they used to be. You may begin to lose your feeling of taste — flavors may not appear as particular to you. Your faculties of smell and contact may likewise debilitate. Your body is taking more time to respond and needs more to invigorate it.

- Your teeth. The intense veneer that shields your teeth from rot can begin to erode throughout the years, leaving you vulnerable to pits. Gum infection is likewise a concern for more established grown-ups. Great dental cleanliness can ensure your teeth and gums. Dry mouth, which is a typical symptom of numerous meds that seniors take, may likewise be an issue.

- Your skin. With a mature age, your skin loses its versatility and may begin to droop and wrinkle. Notwithstanding, the more you shielded your skin from sun harm and smoking when you were more youthful, the better your skin will look as you get more established. Start securing your skin presently to forestall further harm, just as skin malignancy.

- Your sexual coexistence. After menopause, when the monthly cycle stops, numerous women experience physical changes like a loss of vaginal oil. Men may encounter erectile brokenness. Fortunately, the two issues can be effectively treated.

Numerous substantial changes are a natural piece of maturing, yet they don't need to back you off. In addition, there's a ton you can do to secure your body and keep it as healthy as could be expected under the circumstances.

Keys to Aging Well

While keeping up your physical health is essential to healthy maturing, it's likewise key to esteem the experience and development you gain with propelling years. Rehearsing healthy propensities for an amazing duration is perfect, yet it's never past the point of no return receive the rewards of taking great consideration of yourself, even as you get more established.

Here are some healthy maturing tips that are a word of wisdom at any phase of life:

- Stay physically dynamic with normal exercise.
- Stay socially dynamic with loved ones and inside your locale.
- Eat a healthy, well-adjusted diet — dump the low-quality nourishment for fiber-rich, low-fat, and low-cholesterol eating.
- Don't disregard yourself: Regular registration with your primary care physician, dental specialist, and optometrist are significantly increasingly significant at this point.
- Take all meds as coordinated by your primary care physician.
- Limit liquor utilization and cut out smoking.
- Get the rest that your body needs.

At long last, dealing with your physical self is fundamental, yet it's significant that you keep an eye on your enthusiastic health also. Receive the benefits of your long life, and appreciate every single day. This is the ideal opportunity to appreciate great health and joy.

1. Eat a Healthy Diet

Great nourishment and sanitation are particularly significant for more established grown-growth. You constantly need to ensure you eat a healthy, adjusted diet. Follow these tips to assist you with settling on astute nourishment decisions and practice safe nourishment dealing with.

2. Stay away from Common Medication Mistakes

Drugs can treat health issues and assist you with carrying on with a long, healthy life. At the point when utilized erroneously, drugs can likewise cause genuine health issues. Utilize these assets to assist you with settling on keen decisions about the remedy and over-the-counter meds you take.

3. Oversee Health Conditions

It is significant that you work with your healthcare supplier to oversee health problems like diabetes, osteoporosis, and hypertension. You need to get familiar with the medications and gadgets used to treat these regular health issues.

4. Get Screened

Health screenings are a significant method to help perceive health issues - at times before you give any indications or side effects. Ask your healthcare supplier which health screenings are directly for you and discover how often you ought to get screened.

5. Be Active

Exercise and physical action can assist you with remaining fit and solid. You ust don't need to go to a rec center to exercise. Converse with your healthcare supplier about safe ways that you can be dynamic. Look at these assets from the FDA and our administration accomplices.

Additionally, There Are Ways To Prevent Age Sagging Which Are:

Unassuming fixing and lifting

Non-intrusive skin fixing methodology These systems are called non-obtrusive on the grounds that they leave your skin unblemished. You won't have a cut injury, cut, or crude skin a while later. You may see some impermanent redness and grow, however that is typically the main sign that you had a technique.

This is what you can anticipate from a non-intrusive skin-fixing method:

- Results: Tend to show up step by step, so they appear to be natural
- Downtime: Little or none
- Colorblind: Safe for individuals of all skin hues
- Body-wide use: Can fix skin pretty much anyplace on your body

Ultrasound Dermatologists are utilizing ultrasound to send heat profound into the skin.

Main concern: The warmth can make your body produce more collagen. With one treatment, a great many people see unobtrusive lifting and fixing inside 2 to a half year. You may get more profit by having extra medicines.

Radiofrequency During this treatment, your dermatologist, puts a gadget against your skin, which warms the tissue underneath.

Main concern: Most individuals have one treatment and feel some fixing immediately. It need some investment for your body to make collagen, so you'll see the best outcomes in around a half year. A few people profit by having more than one treatment.

Laser treatment Some lasers can send heat profoundly into the skin without injuring the top layer of your skin. These lasers are utilized to fix skin everywhere throughout the body and can be particularly useful for fixing free skin on the tummy and upper arms.

Primary concern: You may require 3 to 5 medications to get results, which step by step show up somewhere in the range of 2 and a half years after the last treatment.

Most fixing and lifting without medical procedure

Insignificantly obtrusive skin fixing strategies While these methodologies can give you increasingly observable outcomes, despite everything, they can't give you the aftereffects of a surgery like a facelift, eyelid medical procedure, or neck lift. Negligibly obtrusive skin fixing, notwithstanding, requires less personal time than a medical procedure. It additionally conveys less danger of reactions.

How to Look Younger than Your Age without Botox, Lasers and Surgery Plus Natural Remedies For Skin Sagging

Getting more seasoned is unavoidable in this life. However, you don't need to look your age on the off chance that you would prefer not to. Truth be told, we'd be eager to wager you feel a lot more youthful than the number you call your "age!" If you've been considering how you can look as youthful as you feel,

Ways to Reverse Facial Aging

1. Dispose of crow's feet and articulation lines

To begin with, we generally evaluate a customer's needs since each patient is exceptional, yet much of the time, we would treat crow's feet with an injectable neurotoxin, for example, Botox or Dysport. It's a straightforward, basically effortless infusion that should be possible on a mid-day break. It produces results in around three to five days, and you'll see fewer lines and wrinkles in the treated zone. Furthermore, don't stress overlooking "solidified"— when done appropriately by a specialist injector, regardless you'll have the option to express and move your face. For progressively harmed skin that has extreme wrinkles, we may recommend a dermal filler or laser reemerging.

2. Delete wrinkles, wrinkles, and poor skin quality

There are ways to treat skin quality issues, running from topical creams to insignificantly obtrusive strategies. Contingent upon the patient's needs and objectives, medicinal evaluation items, injectables, substance strips, and laser reemerging are, for the most part, extraordinary approaches to address wrinkles and wrinkles. Restorative evaluation items are thoroughly scientifically tried and have the most significant levels of dynamic fixings, so they're substantially more powerful and compelling than drugstore counterparts. Furthermore, despite the fact that the name sounds lively, substance strips can be very delicate—they help to shed away dry, dead, unpleasant skin to uncover a softer, more splendid, all the more sparkling appearance.

Laser restoring—the more included alternative since it requires a couple of long stretches of vacation—can drastically revive the skin by getting rid of harmed skin cells and animating your body's own natural mending process. Contingent upon your needs, there's very an alternative that accommodates your way of life, spending plan, and time span.

3. Level out hyperpigmentation, melasma, as well as age spots

One of the best medicines for pigmentation is Broadband Light Therapy. It explicitly targets zones of dark-colored and red pigmentation on the skin to make an all the more even skin tone. Likewise, shedding facial medications, for example, the SilkPeel DermalInfusion System—a 3-in-1 gadget that suctions pores, peels the skin with a jewel tip, and injects the skin with hydrating serums—help with stained regions on the face, neck, and chest. Finally, miniaturized scale needling with PRP (platelet-rich plasma) animates cell turnover and mixes the skin with your body's own mending development factors from your own blood plasma. The outcomes can be truly stunning.

Shining outcomes from a compound strip.

4. Take out your twofold jawline

A twofold jaw can cause you to seem heavier and more seasoned than you are. There are non-obtrusive arrangements that should be possible on a mid-day break, for example, Kybella, an injectable arrangement that disintegrates fat cells, and CoolSculpting. Both of these are generally simple, short-recuperation strategies that our patients love for their benefit and extraordinary outcomes. For a few, Liposuction is a progressively successful alternative, particularly for those with bigger territories of difficult fat.

5. Fix sagging facial skin

As we grow older, our skin lose its versatility and hang, particularly in the lower segment of the face and around the eyes. Often, dermal fillers can assist full with increasing regions that have lost volume, (for example, the sanctuaries, and cheeks), serving to re-form the state of the face and, along these lines, reposition the skin. For other patients with increasingly emotional skin flexibility issues, medical procedures might be the best alternative to address their issues, for example, a facelift, browlift, or eyelid lift.

Facelift results.

6. Peel and see your skin gleam

Customary peeling is significant to keep your skin looking revived. CPS specialists suggest a peeling chemical and standard shedding facial medicines for your best outcome. Facial medicines are profoundly redone to every patient's needs, so your treatment will be customized. Nonetheless, a few top choices are the SilkPeel Dermal Infusion treatment (which feels astounding) and a Dermaplaning Facial during which your skin is delicately shed with a careful cutting edge explicitly intended for evacuating dead skin cells and peach fluff. With both of these alternatives, your skin will be gleaming a while later, and you can approach your day by day standard as expected after the treatment.

7. Restore your skin over a long end of the week

Pass on, in case you're searching for a huge change to your skin, and the Sciton Halo Laser is your long-end of the week saint. It consolidates two laser wavelengths, ablative and non-ablative, into one treatment. That implies you get the noteworthy reemerging of an ablative laser yet with the decreased discomfort and vacation of a non-ablative laser. It's additionally one of the most adjustable laser medicines accessible; settings can be changed so explicitly that CPS can meet exceptionally itemized patient objectives.

8. Stout up your cheeks

As our faces age, the fat cushions in our cheeks and underneath our eyes wither a long time before the face starts to list. On the other way that you are up for some semi-careful work, consider boosting the volume in your cheeks with infusions of hyaluronic corrosive based gel (takes minutes, keeps going eight a year,

9. Have your eyebrows formed

Having your eyebrows formed – and potentially tinted – is one of those minor excellence disclosures that makes you wonder how you at any point got by without it before.

10. Get an extraordinary hairstyle

Having your haircut can be sufficient to make you look years more youthful, and a periphery shrouds a large number of grimace lines. Restorative specialists will often send would-be customers off for a makeover; regularly, and a hairstyle will give them enough certainty to avoid the surgical tool.

11. Sprinkle out on a laser treatment

Almost negligible differences and age spots can both be softened by treatment with fragmentary lasers (the "partial" piece implies that between each gap in the skin made by pinpoint laser bars, there stays a small amount of entire skin that empowers quicker recuperating).

12. Invest energy doing things that satisfy you

You'll feel much improved and look better subsequently. Furthermore, in a similar vein, attempt to grin more. It's more pleasant for every other person, and it fools the body into changing its state of mind. It additionally utilizes fewer muscles than scowling.

13. Cut down on liquor

In addition to the fact that drink has a getting dried out impact on the body, yet it expands the vessels, which prompts a blushing flush on the face (not positively) and has a general provocative impact on the body that empowers maturing.

It's turf's law, yet on the off chance that you lose enough weight to have an obvious effect to the size of your stomach and hips, the other spot where the loss will truly show is in your face. You would prefer not to wind up looking skinny – even the word is maturing.

14. Practice unwinding

We're all super-bustling these days, which raises feelings of anxiety, which is maturing in itself. Unwinding is a propensity that can be educated. Requiring some investment, watching the mists, rehearsing profound breathing – will all assistance facilitate the lines of pressure and stress that settle in through propensity and afterward become a lasting piece of the scene of our appearances.

15. Find the enchantment of medium-term face-promoters

16. Try not to diet too strenuously

17. Brighten your teeth

18. Take the homegrown course to health

How to Get Into Ketosis for Longevity for Women Over 50 Intermittent Fasting On a Keto Diet

Observing One's State Of Ketosis

The ketogenic diet (KD) is an extremely low-starch, high-fat, and satisfactory protein diet with no calorie limit that instigates a metabolic condition called "physiological ketosis." It was first acquainted with treat epilepsy during the 1920s and has become very well known as of late as weight-loss and performance-upgrading diet. Its therapeutic use in the scope of ailments is under scrutiny. During KD mediations, individuals should screen consistent with the dietary routine by day by day pee testing for ketosis.

Discoveries

Twelve healthy subjects (37 ± 11 years; BMI = 23.0 ± 2.5 kg/m2) were told to, during the 6th seven day stretch of a KD and with stable ketosis, measure their pee ($8\times$) and blood ($18\times$) ketone fixation at normal interims during a 24-h period. As indicated by their 1-day nourishment record, the subjects devoured by and large a diet with 74.3 ± 4.0 %, 19.5 ± 3.5 %, and 6.2 ± 2.0 % of absolute vitality consumption from fat, protein, and starch, separately. The most reduced blood ß-hydroxybutyrate (BHB) (0.33 ± 0.17 mmol/l) and pee acetoacetate (AA) (0.46 ± 0.54 mmol/l) fixations were estimated at

10:00, separately. The most elevated BHB (0.70 ± 0.62 mmol/l) and AA focuses were noted at 03:00, separately. By means of pee testing, the most significant levels of ketosis were found at 22:00 and 03:00, and the most noteworthy recognition rates (>90 %) for ketosis were at 07:00, 22:00, and 03:00, individually.

During ketosis, your body changes over fat into mixes known as ketones and starts utilizing them as its principal wellspring of vitality.

Studies have proven to us that diets that advance ketosis are exceptionally useful for weight loss, due to some extent to their craving stifling impacts Emerging examination recommends that ketosis may likewise be useful for type 2 diabetes and neurological issue, among other conditions, Accomplishing a condition of ketosis can take some work and arranging. It's not similarly as straightforward as cutting carbs.

Limit Your Carb Consumption

Eating a low-carb diet is, by a long shot, the most significant factor in accomplishing ketosis.

Regularly, your cells use glucose, or sugar, as their primary wellspring of fuel. Be that as it may, the larger part of your cells can likewise maintain other fuel sources. This includes unsaturated fats, just as ketones, which are otherwise called ketone bodies.

Body keeps glucose in your liver and muscles as glycogen.

When carb admission is exceptionally low, glycogen stores are diminished, and levels of the hormone insulin decrease. This allows unsaturated fats to be discharged from fat stores in your body.

Your liver believers a portion of these unsaturated fats into the ketone bodies CH3)2CO, acetoacetate, and beta-hydroxybutyrate. These ketones can also be utilized as fuel by segments of the mind. The degree of carb limitation expected to actuate ketosis is, to some degree,, individualized. A few people need to constrain net carbs (all-out carbs short fiber) to 20 grams for every day, while others can accomplish ketosis while eating twice this sum or more.

For this explanation, the Atkins diet determines that carbs be limited to 20 or fewer grams for each day for about fourteen days to ensure that ketosis is accomplished.

After this point, limited quantities of carbs can be added back to your diet bit by bit, as long as ketosis is kept up.

Overweight individuals with type 2 diabetes who constrained carb admission to 21 or fewer grams for every day experienced day by day urinary ketone discharge levels that were multiple times higher than their standard levels.

These carb and ketone ranges are prompted for individuals who need to get into ketosis to advance weight loss, control glucose levels, or lessen coronary illness chance variables.

Interestingly, therapeutic ketogenic diets utilized for epilepsy or as trial malignancy therapy often confine carbs to less than 5% of calories or less than 15 grams for every day to continue drive up ketone levels.

As it may, anybody utilizing the diet for therapeutic purposes should just do as such under the supervision of a medicinal professional.

What Are Intermittent Fasting and Metabolic Autophagy

Intermittent Fasting for Longevity and Performance Your cells are continually observing the supplement status of the cells to decide if to monitor vitality or to advance development. **One of a couples of known methods for expanding life expectancy in practically all species is caloric limitation and vitality deprivation.** This triggers numerous metabolic pathways and procedures that make the creature progressively versatile to ecological stressors and subsequently live more. **The digestion has two sub-classifications or sub-forms called anabolism and catabolism. ** * Anabolism, signifying 'upward' in Greek, depicts the synthesis of organic atoms to develop the new physical issues in the body. * Catabolism, signifying 'descending' in Greek, depicts the separating of natural particles to discharge vitality. This can apply to the breakdown of substantial tissue just as the absorption of nourishment that then gets absorbed into the body through anabolic procedures. Notwithstanding 'Metabolic,' you can likewise discover another word in the title - 'Autophagy,' which makes an interpretation of from Ancient Greek into 'self-eating up' or 'eating of self.' This is integral to the primary act of this book. By keeping up harmony among anabolism and catabolism, you can adequately broaden your life expectancy. The procedure of autophagy involves your healthy cells eating up the old, exhausted, frail ones and changing over them once again into vitality. It's truly your body eating itself and utilizing that to look after homeostasis. There are numerous longevity-boosting benefits to this as outlined in for all intents and purposes every single other species. This book is an assortment of rules about the standards of the anabolic-catabolic cycles with respect to nourishment and exercise. It's certainly not a panacea - an answer or solution for all conditions and conditions. Rather, it's quite a certain convention that shouldn't matter for all circumstances. **Metabolic Autophagy will show you: ** * What expands life expectancy in people and other species * Why there's such a lot of sickness and stoutness in the public arena * How to advance health and longevity with intermittent fasting * What is Autophagy and how it functions * How to age increasingly slow vivacious for a mind-blowing duration * Which nourishments make you live more and fabricate muscle * How the supplement controllers of mTOR, AMPK, sirtuins, FOXO proteins, hormesis and others influence longevity * What are circadian rhythms and how they influence your health * Metabolic Autophagy Foods list and their anabolic-catabolic score * Supplements that help muscle development and longevity * Many additional items and rewards concerning nourishment and exercise swim Land is a top of the line writer, anthropologist, business visionary, superior mentor and a biohacker who expounds on improving health and human performance. This book joins day by day way of life and dietary practices that help to cross the abyss among longevity and elite.

How to Fast Intermittent With Keto Diet

Instructions to Combine the Keto Diet With Intermittent Fasting

Is it true that you are hoping to kick off your weight loss? Joining the famous ketogenic diet with intermittent fasting (IF) can bring about swifter weight decrease and enable your body to turn out to be incredibly proficient at consuming fat. To receive these rewards, you need a decent methodology.

So what's the arrangement?

Continue perusing, and you'll figure out how to bit by bit progress into fasting, make a week after week supper plan with a fasting plan, and make the mentality expected to spur yourself. Besides, an area for how to maintain a strategic distance from the normal entanglements of the diet. On the whole, it begins with the nuts and bolts.

The Fundamentals of Ketogenic Diet

The keto diet is a low cab, high fat, moderate protein eating routine that prepares the body to consume fat as its essential fuel. The procedure starts by eating a keto diet. Since it's so low carb, the body rapidly goes through its glycogen stores. At the point when this occurs, you go into ketosis, a metabolic state wherein your body is forced to begin utilizing fat as its essential vitality source. That normally occurs inside around three days.

Next, It ordinarily takes three a month and a half for the body to finish the move over to utilizing fat for fuel. Now, you're fat adjusted. Thus, whenever you're not eating (fasting), your body consequently takes advantage of your fat stores. That is perhaps the main motivation intermittent fasting and keto go together so well. In any case, there are more reasons and favorable circumstances, so continue perusing!

The Keto Diet Advantage for Intermittent Fasting

Along these lines, this book suggests being on the keto diet for four a month and a half before joining intermittent fasting. Not exclusively will you be better at consuming fat, however, you'll have less yearning. In contemplates, the keto diet was demonstrated to be all the more fulfilling, and individuals experienced less yearning. Moreover, keto additionally exhibited its capacity to save bulk and was best in keeping up your digestion. How's that for motivations to begin the ketogenic diet?

Definition of Intermittent Fasting.

Intermittent fasting otherwise known as (IF) is a cycle of eating that pivots between times of fasting and eating. There are four distinct kinds of intermittent fasting. While each is gainful, it's just an issue of an individual inclination concerning which might be best for you.

Sorts of Intermittent Fasting

This strategy incorporates fasting two days of the week and just devouring 500 calories on those days. The other five days, you would keep on eating your typical, healthy keto diet. Since just 500 calories are distributed on fasting days, you would need to expend nourishments that are high in protein and fat so as to keep you satisfied. Simply be certain that there's a nonfasting day in the middle of the two.

1. Time-Restricted Eating

This fasting strategy has demonstrated to be one of the most mainstream as your fasting window, for the most part, incorporates the time you're dozing. The 16/8 quick implies that you are quick for sixteen hours and eat for eight. In actuality, that may mean eating is just permitted from early afternoon to 8 pm, and after that, the quickstarts until the following day. The extraordinary thing about this strategy is that it doesn't need to be 16/8, you can at present do 14/10 and receive similar rewards.

2. Interchange Day Fasting

Notwithstanding the 5;2 technique and time limitation, this choice enables you to be quick every other day, normally constraining yourself to around 500 calories on fasting days. The nonfasting days you would simply eat ordinarily. This can be an extreme methodology and may make some stop as it tends to be hard to keep up.

3. 24 Hour Fast

I have otherwise called "One Meal a Day" or OMAD for short. This quick is accomplished for an entire 24 hours and is generally just done a few times per week.

Next, to begin fasting, you'll need some inspiration to prop you up.

Keeping up the Motivation

Staying with an eating and fasting plan can be intense on the off chance that you come up short on the inspiration – so how might you keep it up? The accompanying focuses will assist keep with concentrating on your general objectives while giving fundamental motivations en route.

PART THREE

Best Exercises For Women Over 50 Tips For Start A Routine At 50+ Weight Loss Tips And Tricks

Quality preparation builds your muscle quality and improves your versatility.

Despite the fact that cardio is very significant for heart and lung health, it's anything but an incredible method to get more fit and keep it off.

At the point when you quit doing a lot of cardio, the weight will rapidly return. Having cardio as a component of your general wellness routine is an unquestionable requirement; be that as it may, quality preparing ought to be the principal factor when you hit the exercise center. Quality preparing expands your muscle quality, yet it will improve your portability, and it is likewise the main thing (alongside appropriate supplements) known to build bone thickness.

In any case, do comprehend that it might appear to be more enthusiastically to pick up muscle as you age because of hormone changes, age-related sickness, and even social variables like a bustling timetable.

As he would like to think, cardio will consume off fat, yet to construct durable muscles, pick substantial weights with few reps or lighter weights with more reps. Likewise, recollect diet and exercise go connected at the hip for generally speaking health and quality, particularly as the year's tick by.

Weight-bearing exercises help with building and keeping up bulk, just as building bone quality and diminishing your hazard for osteoporosis.

"Numerous individuals over [the age of] 50 will quit practicing routinely because of torment in their joints or back or damage, yet don't surrender! Locate a professional that can help get you in the groove again, and expect to get in any event 150 minutes of physical movement [in] seven days to help keep up your bulk and a healthy weight.

1. Try not to skip meals.

As women grow older age, their hormones change, "Estrogen and testosterone progressively decline after some time, which prompts fat collection because of the body not preparing sugar, too. We additionally lose more bulk as we age, causing our resting metabolic rate to diminish. Be that as it may, skipping meals can make you lack in significant key supplements required as we age, for example, by and large calories and protein. Eating normally for the duration of the day and getting enough calories/protein will help with higher vitality levels and keep up bulk, which implies a better ability to burn calories."

Rather, he says it's alright to eat under three meals per day, yet make certain to remain hydrated with a lot of liquids, similar to water, coffee, or tea.

2. Ensure that you get enough rest.

"Perhaps the greatest objection of those over [the age of] 50 is an absence of rest," notes Amselem.

"Rest is vital to healthy weight since two hormones, leptin, and ghrelin, are discharged during rest, and they assume a significant job in craving guidelines. Absence of rest disturbs the procedure and causes metabolic brokenness in which the body befuddles weakness [with] hunger—not something worth being thankful for! My proposal is to get seven to eight hours of rest and, if necessary, take low measurements of melatonin for help."

3. Relinquish old "rules" about weight loss and develop an outlook of health.

"Age impacts weight loss for the two women and men, and that is on the grounds that digestion backs off, hormone levels decay, in addition to there is a loss of bulk,"

"However, that doesn't imply that getting more fit over age [the age of] 50 is mission inconceivable. Diet and exercise are vital; notwithstanding, the basic mix-up I see is that individuals eat and turn out in the equivalent careful manner [that] they [did] when they were more youthful and marvel why they don't get results. Those over [the age of] 50 can't eat and prepare similarly, they did when they were 30. You need to move to get results."

Fortunately, diet and exercise changes are by and large inside your control, says Dr. Ayoob. Make continuous acclimations to advance adjusted eating, rather than falling prey to craze diets, and help yourself to remember the benefits of exercise for your heart, stomach related tract, and psychological wellness, notwithstanding weight the executives.

Make a mentality of wellbeing, prompts Vercelletto. Being over [the age of] 50 isn't a capital punishment—truth be told, a significant number of us presently have more opportunity to deal with ourselves. Having a healthy weight, eating appropriately, not smoking, and constraining liquor utilization is all excessively significant. We are not getting any more youthful, yet we ain't dead yet.

PART FOUR

Keto Meal Ideas, Keto Shopping List Bonus Recipes

(COMPARISM BETWEEN FAST, BEGINNER, ADVANCED, MONTE-TIME SAVING RECIPES)

A Keto Diet Meal Plan for women above 5o+ years and Menu That Can change Your Body

The keto diet, generally speaking, is low in carbs, high in fat and moderate in protein.

When following a ketogenic diet, carbs are regularly diminished to under 50 grams for every day, however stricter and looser adaptations of the diet exist.

Fats ought to supplant most of the cut carbs and convey roughly 75% of your all-out calorie consumption.

Proteins should symbolise around 20% of vitality needs, while carbs are generally limited to 5%.

This carb decrease forces your body to depend on fats for its primary vitality source to glucose — a procedure known as ketosis.

While in ketosis, your body utilizes ketones — particles delivered in the liver from fats when glucose is restricted — as another fuel/enrgy source.

Despite the fact that fat is often maintained a strategic distance from for its unhealthy substance, explore shows that ketogenic diets are fundamentally more powerful at advancing weight loss than low-fat diets

In addition, keto diets decrease yearning and increment satiety, which can be especially useful when attempting to get in shape.

Ketogenic Diet Meal Plan

Exchanging over to a ketogenic diet can show to be overpowering, yet it doesn't need to be troublesome.

Your attention ought to be on decreasing carbs while expanding the fat and protein substance of meals and bites.

In other reach and stay in a condition of ketosis, carbs must be limited.

While certain individuals may just accomplish ketosis by eating under 20 grams of carbs every day, others might be fruitful with a lot higher carb admission.

By and large, the lower your sugar admission, the simpler it is to reach and remain in ketosis.

This is the reason adhering to keto-accommodating nourishments and maintaining a strategic distance from things rich in carbs is the ideal approach to get thinner on a ketogenic diet effectively.

Keto-Friendly Foods to Eat

When following a ketogenic diet, meals and bites should base on the accompanying nourishments:

- Eggs: Pastured, entire natural eggs settle on the best decision.
- Poultry: Chicken and turkey.
- Fatty fish: Wild-got salmon, herring, and mackerel.
- Meat: Grass-nourished hamburger, venison, pork, organ meats, and buffalo.
- Full-fat dairy: Yogurt, margarine, and cream.
- Full-fat cheddar: Cheddar, mozzarella, brie, goat cheddar, and cream cheddar.
- Nuts and seeds: Macadamia nuts, almonds, pecans, pumpkin seeds, peanuts, and flaxseeds.
- Nut margarine: Natural nut, almond, and cashew spreads.
- Fats: Coconut oil, olive oil, avocado oil, coconut margarine, and sesame oil.
- Avocados: Whole avocados can be added to practically any feast or bite.
- Non-boring vegetables: Greens, broccoli, tomatoes, mushrooms, and peppers.
- Condiments: Salt, pepper, vinegar, lemon juice, crisp herbs and flavors.

Nourishments to Avoid

Stay away from nourishments rich in carbs while following a keto diet.

The accompanying nourishments ought to be confined:

- Bread and heated merchandise: White bread, entire wheat bread, wafers, treats, doughnuts, and rolls.
- Sweets and sugary nourishments: Sugar, frozen yogurt, sweet, maple syrup, agave syrup, and coconut sugar.
- Sweetened refreshments: Soda, juice, improved teas, and sports drinks.
- Pasta: Spaghetti and noodles.
- Grains and grain items: Wheat, rice, oats, breakfast oats
- Starchy vegetables: Potatoes, sweet potatoes, butternut squash, corn, peas, and pumpkin.
- Beans and vegetables: Black beans, chickpeas, lentils, and kidney beans.
- Fruit: Citrus, grapes, bananas and pineapple.
- High-carb sauces: Barbecue sauce, a sugary serving of mixed greens dressings, and plunging sauces.
- Certainly mixed refreshments: Beer and sugary blended beverages.

Despite the fact that carbs ought to be confined, low-glycemic organic products, for example, berries can be delighted in constrained sums insofar as you're keeping up a keto-accommodating macronutrient extend.

Make certain to pick healthy nourishment sources and avoid prepared food sources and unhealthy fats.

The accompanying things ought to be stayed away from:

- Unhealthy fats: Margarine, shortening, and vegetable oils, for example, canola and corn oil.

- Processed nourishments: Fast nourishment, bundled food sources, and prepared meats, for example, wieners and lunch meats.

- Diet nourishments: Foods that contain counterfeit hues, additives and sugars, for example, sugar alcohols and aspartame.

A Sample Keto Menu for One Week

The accompanying menu gives under 50 grams of complete carbs every day.

As referenced above, a few people may need to decrease starches much further so as to arrive at ketosis.

General one-week ketogenic menu that can be changed, relying upon singular dietary needs.

Monday

- Breakfast: Two eggs seared in fed margarine presented with sauteed greens.
- Lunch: A bunless grass-encouraged burger beat with cheddar, mushrooms, and avocado on a bed of greens.
- Dinner: Pork hacks with green beans sauteed in coconut oil.

Tuesday

- Breakfast: Mushroom omelet.

- Lunch: Tuna plate of mixed greens with celery and tomato on a bed of greens.
- Dinner: Roast chicken with cream sauce and sauteed broccoli.

Wednesday

- Breakfast: Bell pepper loaded down with cheddar and eggs.
- Lunch: Arugula plate of mixed greens with hard-bubbled eggs, turkey, avocado, and blue cheddar.
- Dinner: Grilled salmon with spinach sauteed in coconut oil.

Thursday

- Breakfast: Full-fat yogurt bested with Keto granola.
- Lunch: Steak bowl with cauliflower rice, cheddar, herbs, avocado, and salsa.
- Dinner: Bison steak with gooey broccoli.

Friday

- Breakfast: Baked avocado egg pontoons.
- Lunch: Caesar serving of mixed greens with chicken.
- Dinner: Pork cleaves with vegetables.

Saturday

- Breakfast: Cauliflower toast beat with cheddar and avocado.
- Lunch: Bunless salmon burgers beat with pesto.
- Dinner: Meatballs presented with zucchini noodles and parmesan cheddar.

Sunday

- Breakfast: Coconut milk chia pudding beat with coconut and pecans.
- Lunch: Cobb serving of mixed greens made with greens, hard-bubbled eggs, avocado, cheddar, and turkey.
- Dinner: Coconut chicken curry.

As should be obvious, ketogenic meals can be assorted and tasty.

Albeit numerous ketogenic meals are based around creature items, there is a wide assortment of veggie lover alternatives to browse also.

KETO CHAFFLE RECIPES 2020

100+ Mouth Watering Low Carb Recipes For
Beginners. Bonus: Gluten Free Recipes For Athletes
+ Anti Aging Recipes For Women Over 50 +
Ketogenic Diet Cookbook

Serena Green

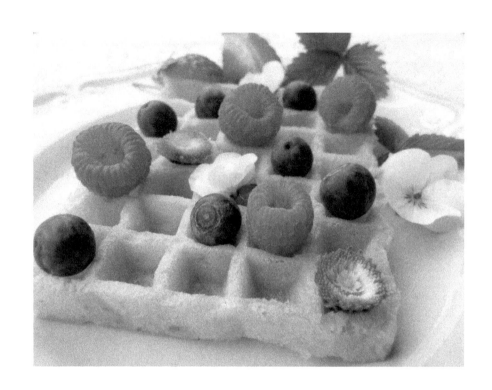

The Meaning Of Chaffle

Chaffles (short for cheddar waffles) are the most recent famous nourishment in the keto world. It's nothing unexpected — the chaffle has a great deal putting it all on the line. This straightforward keto formula is fresh, brilliant dark colored, sans sugar, low-carb, and exceptionally simple to make.

A chaffle, or cheddar waffle, is a keto waffle made with eggs and cheddar. Chaffles are turning into an extremely well known keto/low-carb nibble.

A chaffle is a waffle yet made with a cheddar base. Basically it's obliterated cheddar and an egg mix. Once in for a short time for logically fluffier recipes, it's a cream cheddar base instead of decimated cheddar. It's the a la mode new keto-pleasing bread since it's low in carbs, and it won't spike your insulin levels, causing fat accumulating.

The fundamentals are some combo of egg and cheddar; however, from here, you can riff like wild eyed. You can use an arrangement of cheeses, including cream cheddar, parmesan cheddar, etc. Some incorporate almond flour and flaxseed and getting ready powder, and others don't.

The major recipe for a chaffle contains cheddar, almond flour, and an egg. You consolidate the fixings in an astonish and pour it your waffle maker. Waffle makers are no doubt on the rising right now after this chaffle recipe exploded a couple of days back earlier. I was to some degree suspicious from the beginning intuition there was no possibility this would turn out in the wake of joining everything and pouring the hitter over the waffle. Try to sprinkle the waffle maker really well. The waffle wound up exceptional, and it was firm apparently and fragile in the inside.

You can concoct a chaffle utilizing a waffle iron or smaller than usual waffle producer. The cook time is just a couple of moments, and on the off chance that you cook the chaffle right, you end up with a fresh, gooey, flavorful bread/waffle elective.

Chaffles are turning into somewhat of a furor with supporters of the keto diet. They're less fastidious to make than most keto bread recipes and they're anything but difficult to customize. You can transform the fundamental formula for a chaffle into your own creation, running from flavorful to sweet and anything in the middle. You can likewise change the sort of cheddar you use, delivering significant changes in the flavor and surface of the chaffle. Cheddar and mozzarella cheddar are the two most regular decisions, yet you can likewise include parmesan, cream cheddar, or whatever other cheddar that melts well.

The most fundamental clarification of a Chaffle is that it's an extraordinary bread elective when on the keto diet. It copies the vibe of a waffle however Keto clients have been utilizing Chaffles in a wide range of recipes from sandwiches to sweets. There are a huge amount of Keto Chaffle Recipes out there.

The first chaffle formula starting point is obscure. Be that as it may, what a chaffle is – well, it's Keto enchantment in your mouth. It's a low carb waffle that works AWESOME for filling your requirement for bread. It just takes a couple of fixings, can be made in merely minutes and is made in a waffle creator.

It's made with cheddar, so get it? At the point when you work cheddar and waffle – you get chaffle (and you additionally get enchantment.) Well enough with the back story. Since you realize what this keto nourishment is, how about we make one and let you see with your own eyes how astounding this keto waffle is.

What Is Needed To Prepare A Chaffle

- 1 tremendous egg
- 1/2 c. Cheddar
- 2 tablespoons of almond flour

How To Prepare A Chaffle

There are a few hints, techniques and approaches you'll need to know to make your chaffles particularly fresh.

Most importantly, don't eat your chaffles directly out of the waffle iron. They'll be wet and eggy from the outset, however on the off chance that you let them sit for 3-4 minutes, they'll fresh right up.

Second, for extra fresh chaffles, you can include an additional layer of destroyed cheddar (or another cheddar that gets firm, similar to parmesan) to the two sides of the waffle producer's surface. Set out the destroyed cheddar, pour in the hitter, put more cheddar on top, and afterward cook the chaffle typically. You'll wind up with firm, sautéed bits of cheddar installed in the outside of the chaffle.

Everyone is going looney tunes, asking, "How might I make these?!" This is the game plan The principal recipe on what and how. The fundamental equation consolidates crushed cheddar and an egg; however, there are tremendous measures of add-ins you can use to change the flavor! You will make a direct chaffle hitter and cook it in a waffle maker!

To make a chaffle equation, you will fundamentally join two or three fixings and cook it in a waffle maker to make a perfect work of art everyone will value!

1. Preheat your waffle maker if it requires preheating.
2. Whisk together the egg, cheddar, almond flour, and setting up the soda pop in a bowl until all-around joined.
3. Shower the waffle maker with a cooking sprinkle and pour the chaffle player over the waffle maker. Close and let the waffle for 3 to 4 minutes. My waffle maker has it's own customized clock setting.
4. Remove the waffle from the waffle press and welcome it.

The Waffle Tools To Make Easy Keto Chaffles

A standard waffle creator will deliver a chaffle that appears as though the universally adored round solidified toaster waffles, which is flawless as keto bread for sandwiches, a bun for burgers, or even a shell for tacos. One famous brand is the Dash smaller than expected waffle creator, which is entirely reasonable and makes slender, fresh chaffles.

A Belgian waffle creator makes thicker waffles with profound scores. That is incredible for typical waffle-production, however it isn't perfect for chaffles. They end up less fresh, with a greater amount of an omelet-like consistency. Your most logical option is to get a standard waffle producer.

How To Eat Chaffles

There are a great deal of famous approaches to eat chaffles.

- Plain. Chaffles are incredible all alone as a morning meal nourishment. You can serve them up close by bacon, eggs, avocado, and other standard keto breakfast passage.

- Keto chaffle sandwich. Make two chaffles and use them as bread for your preferred sandwich. Chaffles are extraordinary as the bread for BLTs, turkey clubs, breakfast sandwiches, or some other keto-accommodating sandwich.

- Chaffle dessert. Attempt one of the sweet chaffle varieties recorded underneath and present with keto maple syrup or your most loved keto frozen yogurt.

The Different Type Of Waffle Maker Needed To Make A Chaffle

By far most genuinely like to use a Dash Mini Waffle Maker; however, you can use any waffle maker you have. There is a wide scope of waffle makers. Honestly, you in all likelihood have one in the back of your kitchen organizers that you haven't used in quite a while. Most by far who don't have a waffle maker may even find one at a Goodwill or Salvation Army. There's no absence of these helpful kitchen gadgets in these reused stores.

The Various Types Of Basic Keto Chaffle Recipes

Keto Chaffle Recipes eBook Cookbook for beginners 2020, includes delicious and appealing keto recipes for each flavor palette.

1. Basic Chaffle Recipes
2. Savory Chaffle Recipes

3. Sweet Chaffle Recipes
4. Chaffle Cake Recipes

Various Cheeses

Cheddar, mozzarella, parmesan, cream cheddar, colby jack — any cheddar that melts well will work with a chaffle. Distinctive cheddar produce various flavors and somewhat various surfaces. Attempt a couple and locate your top choice.

Sweet Chaffles

Utilize a nonpartisan cheddar like mozzarella or cream cheddar, at that point include a touch of your most loved keto sugar to the hitter before you cook it. You can likewise chocolate chips or low-sugar fruits like blueberries or strawberries. Top with keto frozen yogurt or keto whipped cream for a delectable chaffle dessert.

Exquisite Chaffles

Include exquisite fixings like herbs and flavors to your chaffle. For a pizza chaffle, include oregano, garlic powder, and diced pepperoni in the hitter, with tomato sauce and additional cheddar on top. Or on the other hand you could utilize cream cheddar and add everything bagel flavoring to the player for an everything bagel chaffle. Present with more cream cheddar on top, tricks, onions, and smoked salmon.

Rules On How To Make The Best Chaffles

1. Tolerance. That is the best tip. They don't take long, yet if you need a new keto waffle, you are just should be to some degree patient and let it take the 5-7 minutes that it takes to new up. Precisely when you trust it's done? Permit it one greater minute or two. Make an effort not to flood.

2. Layering. In the event that you're making a chaffle with cheddar, the best way to deal with do this is to layer cheddar at the base, pour in a tablespoon or so of egg, and a short time later top with cheddar again. It's the firm cheddar on the base and top that will make them new.

3. Shallow waffles. If you need new waffles, the shallower the waffle iron, the more straightforward/faster it is to new up the chaffle.

4. No over-burdening. Stuffed chaffle makers… well, they flood clearly. Which makes colossal destruction! So when in doubt, under fill rather than pressing. Near 1/4 cup of TOTAL fixings in a steady progression.

5. Crush it. I've thought about others using press bottles so they can get just a little egg into the small scale waffle maker.

6. Simple cleanup. I like to use a wet paper towel when the waffle iron is warm, to make cleanup straightforward. Not hot, however, obviously! Essentially warm.

7. Brush it. I've found toothbrush works outstandingly to clean between the waffle iron teeth. You can in like manner endeavor this wipe cleaner, which I also use to clean the little region on the edge of my Instant Pot.

8. No looking. I can tell you from LOTS of individual experience, that opening the waffle iron at normal interims "just to check" doesn't hep the chaffle cook any speedier. Your most consistent choice is to not using any and all means open it for 4-5 minutes.

9. No steaming. on the off chance that you're using the Dash small, the little blue light goes out when it's commonly cooked, yet most importantly, the chaffle stops steaming to such a degree. That is a better than average sign that it's done.

10. Get hot. Hold up until the waffle iron is hot before you incorporate fixings, and they're essentially less slanted to adhere and a lot easier to clean up.

11. Tangle it. Alright, so about that flood. I do find that it unfolds more routinely than I may need! One thing that has made cleanup more straightforward for me has been to put a silicone trivet underneath.

12. Cut or shred. I understand most recipes out there suggest demolished cheddar, yet I have better karma with the slimmest cut of cheddar I can buy. I find it crisps essentially speedier.

13. Not really eggy. If you find your chaffles too eggy, use egg white as opposed to the whole egg.

14. Not really gooey. In case you need them to taste less gooey, endeavor mozzarella cheddar.

15. Fresh Cooling. License the chaffles to cool before eating. They get crisper as they cool, so take the necessary steps not to stuff the hot chaffle into your mouth right away.

16. Make parts. Make enough to share, and everyone will require them, whether or not they're keto or not.

Chaffles Nutrition and Carb Count

You'll get two chaffles out of an enormous egg and about a large portion of a cup of cheddar. Contingent upon the cheddar you use, your calories and net carb check will change a tad. Yet, as a rule, expecting you utilize genuine, entire milk cheddar like cheddar or mozzarella (rather than cream cheddar or American cheddar), chaffles are totally sans carb. A normal serving size of two chaffles contains generally:

- 300 calories
- 0g all out carbs
- 0g net carbs
- 20g protein
- 23g fat

As should be obvious, chaffles are about as keto as a formula can be: high-fat, high-protein, and zero-carb. They even work on the flesh eater diet, if you eat cheddar.

The Best Keto Chaffle Recipes To Try

Including recipes for some work of art, high-carb top picks that have been adjusted to be "fat bombs," which help keep your macros in balance, just as keep you from desiring every one of the things you, for the most part, can't eat when you're attempting to get more fit.

A considerable amount of the in excess of 200 recipes require close to 10 to 15 minutes of planning time, and they taste as scrumptious and liberal as they sound–what about Chocolate Peanut Butter Pops, Mocha Cheesecake, or Almond Butter Bombs?

Keto Chaffle Recipe

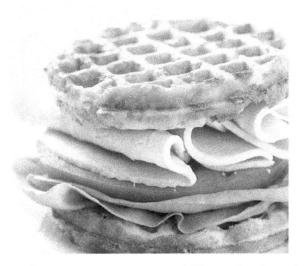

Keto chaffles are the most recent new rage! The entire formula is just 3 net carbs all out.

Ingredients

- 1 huge egg
- 1/2 c. Cheddar
- 2 tablespoons of almond flour

Rich And Creamy Chaffles Recipe

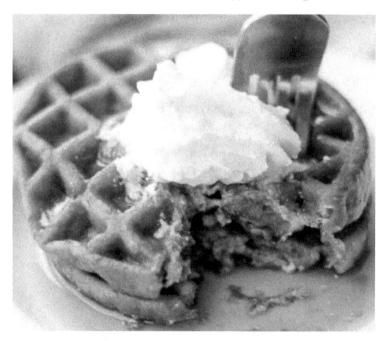

- 2 eggs
- 1 cup destroyed mozzarella
- 2 tablespoons almond flour
- 2 tablespoons cream cheddar
- 3/4 Tbsp. preparing power
- 3 tablespoons water (discretionary)

- Makes 6 waffles.

Zucchini Chuffles | Zuffles Recipe

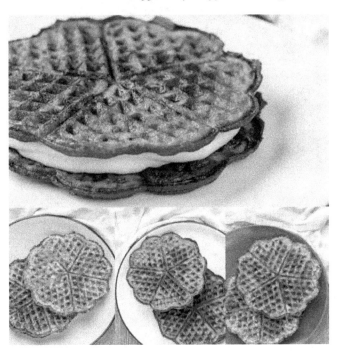

- 1 little zucchini, ground
- 1 egg
- 1 tablespoon parmesan
- Small bunch of destroyed mozzarella
- Basil and pepper to taste
- Mix all together and cook in a full-size waffle producer.
- Makes 2 full-size waffles and a meager zaffle.

Light And Crispy Chaffles Recipe

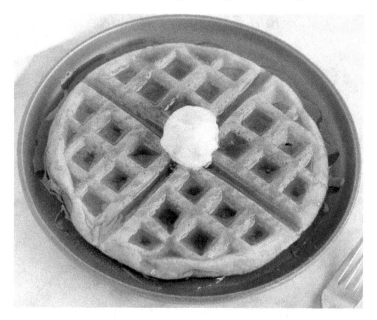

- 1 egg

- 1/3 cup cheddar

- 1/4 Tbsp. heating powder

- 1/2 Tbsp. ground flaxseed

- Shredded parmesan cheddar on top and base.

- Stir and cook in a mini waffle iron until fresh.

Keto Sausage Ball

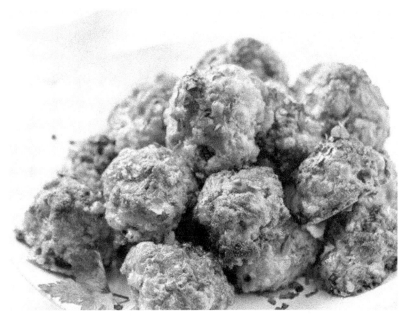

Portrayal

Keto Sausage Balls just contain four straightforward ingredients and make an extraordinary canapé or bite. They just contain 1 net carb and can without much of a stretch fit into your low carb or keto way of life.

Ingredients

- 2 cups of almond flour

2 Cups Of Cheddar

- 1 pound of pork wiener
- 8 oz of cream cheddar

Fat Head Pizza Crust

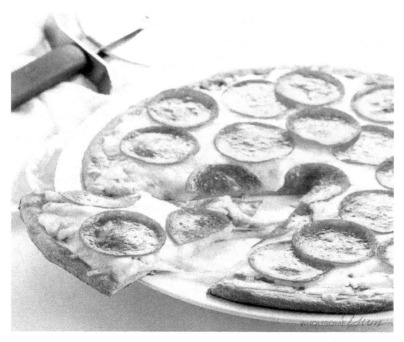

Ingredients

- 1 1/2 cups destroyed mozzarella
- 3/4 cup almond flour
- 2 tablespoons of cream cheddar, cubed
- 1 egg
- garlic powder, onion powder, and blended herbs for flavoring *see notes

Chicken Stuffed Avocado

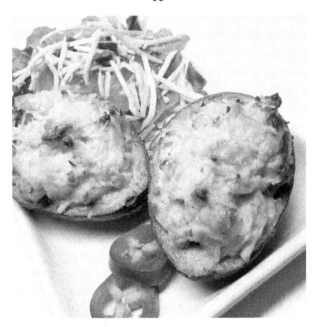

Portrayal

Wild ox Chicken Stuffed Avocado is a brisk formula utilizing stovetop bison chicken plunge and avocados. Making wild ox chicken plunge is extremely simple utilizing a stovetop too.

Ingredients

- 2 5 oz jars of chicken, depleted
- 2 tablespoons of whipped cream cheddar
- 2 tsp of dry Ranch flavoring blend
- ¼ cup of sans fat cheddar (utilize full fat with keto or low carb)
- 2 tablespoons of Frank's Buffalo Wing Sauce
- 1 medium avocado

Almond Flour Blueberry Pancakes

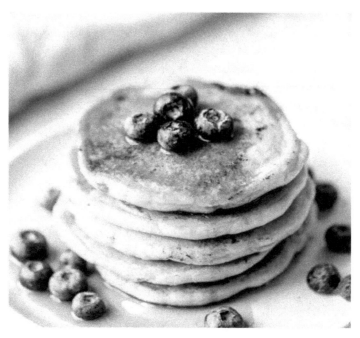

Depiction

Basic almond flour flapjacks made with just 6 ingredients. 2 net carbs per hotcake!

Ingredients

- 2 huge eggs
- ⅓ cup unsweetened almond milk
- 1 Tbsp. vanilla concentrate
- 1 ¼ cup fine almond flour (utilized Bob's, Red Mill)
- ¼ Tbsp. preparing pop
- Touch of salt
- Spread for lubing the skillet

Boston Brown Bread Recipe

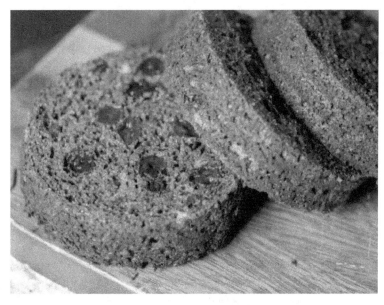

Ingredients

- 1 Egg
- 1 cup buttermilk, or 1 cup milk with 1 tablespoon vinegar blended in
- 1/4 cup Molasses
- 1/4 cup Sugar
- 1 tablespoon Oil
- 1.5 cups Whole Wheat Flour
- 1/2 cup Cornmeal
- 2 Tbsp.s Baking Powder
- 1 Tbsp. Ground Allspice
- 1/2 cup slashed pecans

- 1/4 cup Raisins

Keto Cheese Muffins

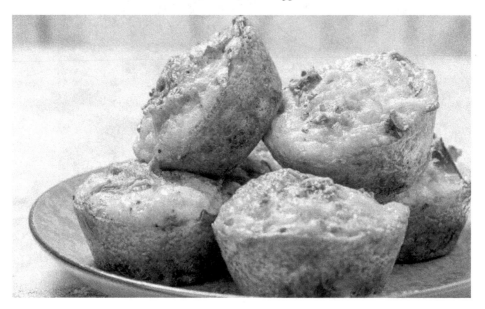

Ingredients

- Vegetable oil for lubing the skillet
- 1 cup (112 g) Superfine Almond Flour
- 1/2 cup (85 g) Black Chia Seeds
- 2 Tbsp.s (2 Tbsp.s) Baking Powder
- 1/2 Tbsp. (118.29 g) granulated garlic
- 4 enormous (4 huge) Eggs
- 1/4 cup (56.75 g) softened margarine
- 1/2 cup (56.5 g) ground cheddar

Air Fryer Breaded Chicken Wings

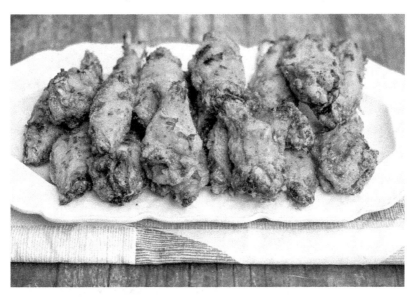

Ingredients

- 1 pound (453.59 g) chicken wings
- 3 tablespoons (3 tablespoons) Vegetable Oil
- 1/2 cup (62.5 g) All-Purpose Flour
- 1/2 Tbsp. (0.5 Tbsp.) Smoked Paprika
- 1/2 Tbsp. (0.5 Tbsp.s) Garlic Powder
- 1/2 Tbsp. (0.5 Tbsp.) Salt
- 1/2 Tbsp. (0.5 Tbsp.s) naturally squashed peppercorn

One Step Brazilian Pao De Queijo Brazilian Cheese Bread

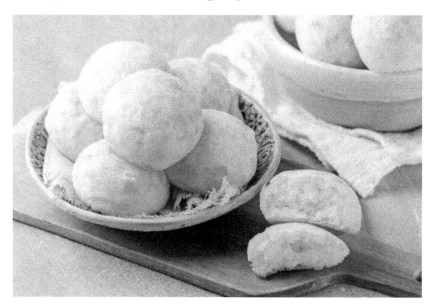

Ingredients

- 1 cup (244 g) Whole Milk
- 1/2 cup (112 g) Oil
- 1 Tbsp. (1 Tbsp.) Salt
- 2 cups (240 g) Tapioca Flour
- 2 (2) Eggs
- 1.5 cups (150 g) destroyed parmesan cheddar

Keto Zucchini Walnut Bread

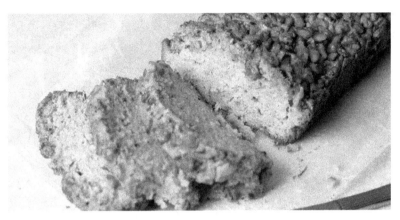

Need to make a Keto Zucchini Bread, you'll be super eager to eat and serve to other people? This formula with pecans is great!

Ingredients

- 1/2 cup (0.5 g) Truvia
- 3 (3) Eggs
- 1/2 cup (109 g) Ghee or Oil
- 1.5 cups (168 g) Superfine Almond Flour
- 1/2 cups (60 g) coconut flour
- 1 Tbsp. (1 Tbsp.) Baking Powder
- 1 Tbsp. (1 Tbsp.) Baking Soda
- 1/2 Tbsp. (0.5 Tbsp.s) Ground Cinnamon
- 1/4 Tbsp. Ground Nutmeg
- 1/2 cup (250 g) Unsweetened Almond Milk
- 2 cups (248 g) destroyed zucchini
- 1 cup (117 g) cleaved pecans

Keto Bread | Nut And Seed Bread

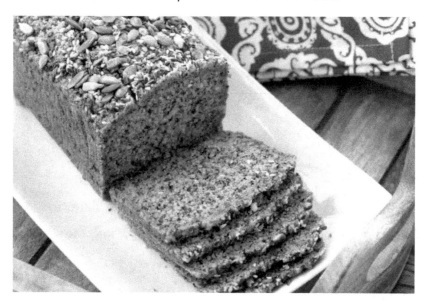

Ingredients

3 cups blended nuts and seeds left entire for instance

- 1/2 cup (61.5 g) pistachios
- 1/2 cup (71.5 g) almonds
- 1/2 cup (84 g) flaxseed
- 1/2 cup (58.5 g) pecans
- 1/2 cup (75 g) Sesame Seeds
- 1/2 cup (64.5 g) cashews

Different INGREDIENTS

- 3 (3) Eggs
- 1/4 cup (56 ml) Oil
- 1/3 tsp (0.33 tsp) Salt

One Step Brazilian Pao De Queijo Brazilian Cheese Bread

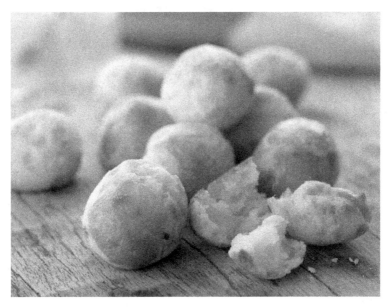

Ingredients

- 1 cup (244 g) Whole Milk
- 1/2 cup (112 g) Oil
- 1 Tbsp. (1 Tbsp.) Salt
- 2 cups (240 g) Tapioca Flour
- 2 (2) Eggs
- 1.5 cups (150 g) destroyed parmesan cheddar

Sweet Cream Truffles

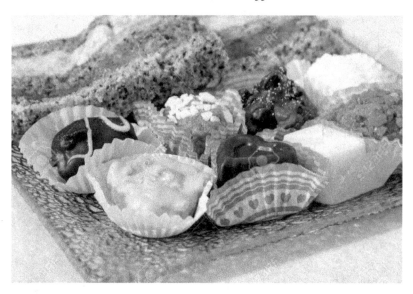

Ingredients

For the Truffle Center

- 2 cups (476 g) Heavy Whipping Cream
- 1/2 cup (91 g) powdered Swerve
- For the Chocolate Coating
- 2 ounces (56.7 g) Sugar-Free Chocolate Chips
- 1 tablespoon (1 tablespoon) Butter

Keto Milky Bears| Gummy Bear Recipe

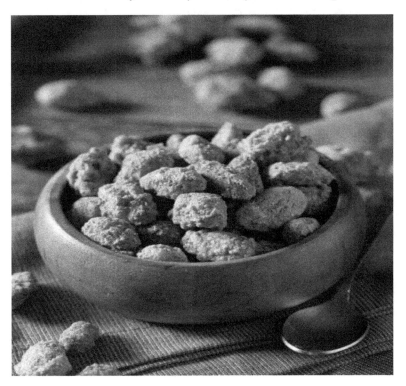

These Keto Milky Bears are a fabulous sweet treat that won't take you out of ketosis. They're low carb, without gluten thus great you can't simply eat one! Obviously superior to normal keto sticky bears.

Ingredients

- 1 13.5 ounces (1) Full-Fat Coconut Milk
- 2 bundles (2) unflavored gelatin, (3 tablespoons)
- 1/4 cup (62.5 g) Water
- 3 tablespoons (3 tablespoons) Truvia
- 2-3 drops (2) Pandan Extract

Keto Coconut Panna Cotta

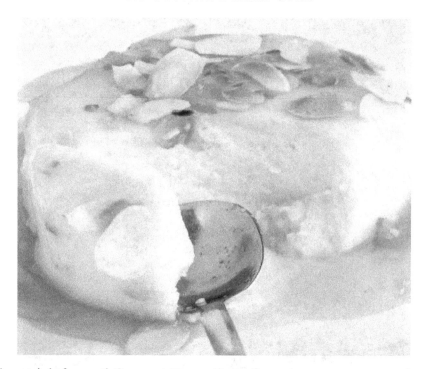

This straightforward Coconut Panna Cotta formula so sweet, smooth, and yummy that it will get one of your go-to pastries! Also, it's low carb and dairy-free!

Ingredients

- 1/2 cup cold water
- 1 bundle unflavored gelatin, 1/4 oz or 2.5 Tbsp.s
- 13.5 ounces Full-Fat Coconut Milk
- 1/8 cup Truvia
- 1 Tbsp. unadulterated vanilla concentrate or coconut extricate

Keto Chocolate Cheesecake Brownies

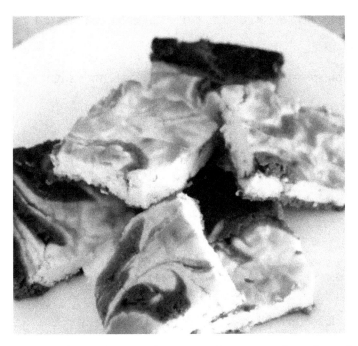

These Keto Chocolate Cheesecake Brownies are a chocolate cheesecake darlings dream! They're so acceptable you won't have the option to tell their low carb!

Ingredients

For the Brownie Batter

- 1/2 cup (90 g) Sugar-Free Chocolate Chips
- 1/2 cup (113.5 g) Butter
- 3 (3) Eggs
- 1/4 cup (0.25 g) Truvia, or other sugar
- 1 Tbsp. (1 Tbsp.) vanilla concentrate

- For the Cheesecake Batter

- 8 ounces (226.8 g) Cream Cheese, cubed and relaxed

- 1 (1) Egg

- 3 tablespoons (3 tablespoons) Truvia, or other sugar

- 1 Tbsp. (1 Tbsp.) vanilla concentrate

Keto Pie Crust

This 3-ingredient pat out Keto Pie Crust formula is a keto dieter's dream! No compelling reason to make crustless pies so as to keep it low carb. It's totally keto and vegan.

Ingredients

- 1 cup (112 g) Superfine Almond Flour

- 2 tablespoons (2 tablespoons) powdered Swerve

- 1/4 cup (54.5 g) Melted Coconut Oil

Keto Maple Pecan Blondies

These Keto Maple Pecan Blondies are the ideal sweet treat to fulfill your sweet tooth. They're wonderfully rich and shockingly low carb!

Ingredients

- 1 cup (112 g) Superfine Almond Flour

- 1/4 cup (30 g) coconut flour

- 2 Tbsp.s (2 Tbsp.s) Baking Powder

- 1/2 cup (91 g) Swerve

- 1/2 cup (113.5 g) Butter, softened

- 3 (3) Eggs
- 1 Tbsp. (1 Tbsp.) maple separate
- 3/4 cup (87.75 g) slashed pecans

Keto Lasagna

Make this simple Keto Lasagna formula in your air fryer utilizing zucchini rather than conventional pasta noodles. It's so acceptable you won't miss the pasta!

Ingredients

- 1 cup marinara sauce
- 1 zucchini, cut into long, flimsy cuts
- For Meat Layer
- 1 cup finely slashed yellow onion
- 1 Tbsp. Minced Garlic
- 1/2 pound-mass hot or mellow Italian frankfurter
- 1/2 cup ricotta cheddar
- 1/2 cup destroyed mozzarella cheddar
- 1/2 cup destroyed parmesan,, isolated
- 1 Egg
- 1/2 Tbsp. Garlic, minced
- 1/2 Tbsp. Italian Seasoning
- 1/2 Tbsp. Ground Black Pepper

Keto Almond Phirni Kheer

This Keto Almond Phirni Kheer is a heavenly Indian pastry formula that you're going to experience passionate feelings for! In addition, it is tasty, it's low carb as well!

Ingredients

- 3/4 cup (178.5 g) Heavy Whipping Cream
- 1 cup (250 g) Unsweetened Almond Milk
- 1/2 cup (56 g) Superfine Almond Flour
- 2 tablespoons (2 tablespoons) Truvia
- 1/2-1 Tbsp. (0.5 Tbsp.s) Ground Cardamom
- 2-3 (2) Saffron Strands, squashed

Tomato Eggplant Soup

This is such an incredible vegan Tomato Eggplant Soup formula! Empty everything into your Instant Pot, and you'll have a bowl of great Mediterranean soup for supper in less than 30 minutes.

Ingredients

- 3 tablespoons Oil
- 2 tablespoons Minced Garlic
- 4 cups Eggplant, hacked
- 2 cups Tomatoes, hacked, or 1 14.5 ounce canned tomatoes, depleted
- 1 cup Onion, hacked

- 1 cup chime pepper, cleaved
- 1/2 cup Water
- 1 Tbsp. salt
- 1 Tbsp. Ground Black Pepper
- For Finishing
- 1/4 cup Basil, hacked

Hamburger Kheema Meatloaf

Tired of normal meatloaf? Can't manage one more night of tacos to go through that ground hamburger? Make proper acquaintance with air fryer keto Indian Kheema meatloaf! Appreciate Indian food in a manner you may be comfortable with by making this Beef Kheema Meatloaf in your Air Fryer.

Ingredients

- 1 lb Lean Ground Beef
- 2 Eggs
- 1 cup Onion, diced
- 1/4 cup Cilantro, hacked
- 1 tbsp minced ginger
- 1 tbsp Minced Garlic
- 2 tsp Garam Masala
- 1 tsp Salt
- 1 tsp Turmeric
- 1 tsp cayenne

- 1/2 tsp Ground Cinnamon
- 1/8 tsp Ground Cardamom

Weight Cooker Low Carb Wontons

Make these low carb wontons in your Instant pot, for the most delicate and succulent low carb wontons you've at any point had. Make these wontons without any wrappers, yet the entirety of the flavor of customary wontons.

Ingredients

- 1 pound (453.59 g) ground pork
- 1/4 cup (25 g) Green Onions, green and white parts blended
- 1/4 cup (4 g) Chopped Cilantro or Parsley
- 2 Tbsp.s (2 Tbsp.s) Soy Sauce
- 1 Tbsp. (1 Tbsp.) Oyster sauce
- 1 Tbsp. (1 Tbsp.) Ground Black Pepper
- ½ Tbsp. (0.5 Tbsp.) Salt
- 1 tablespoon (1 tablespoon) minced ginger
- 1 tablespoon (1 tablespoon) Minced Garlic
- 2 (2) Eggs

Keto Chicken Biryani

This Low Carb Chicken Biryani formula is Low-Carb Indian Food at it's ideal. Cauliflower and ground chicken make up this fiery, heavenly low carb formula.

Ingredients

For Chicken

- 1 Tbsp. Ghee
- 1 pound Ground Chicken
- 1 Tbsp. salt
- 1/2 Tbsp. Turmeric
- 1 Tbsp. Garam Masala
- 1/2 Tbsp. Ground Coriander
- 1/4 Tbsp. Ground Cumin

Vegetables

- 1 Tbsp. Ghee
- 1 Red Onion, cut meager
- 1 Jalapeño pepper, diced
- 1 Tbsp. ginger-garlic glue, (or 1/2 Tbsp.s minced garlic, 1/2 Tbsp.s minced ginger)
- 1/2 cup Water
- 1/2 cup Cilantro, slashed
- 1/4 cup mint leaves, slashed
- 2 cups cauliflower, riced

Moment Pot Cauliflower "Macintosh" And Cheese Low Carb

Moment Pot Low Carb Keto Cauliflower and Cheese is a velvety, delightful side dish that you can make in your weight cooker for a definitive low carb comfort food!

Ingredients

- 2 cups (214 g) cauliflower, riced
- 2 tablespoon (2 tablespoons) Cream Cheese
- 1/2 cup (56.5 g) destroyed sharp cheddar
- 1/2 Tbsp. (0.5 Tbsp.) Salt
- 1/2 Tbsp. (0.5 Tbsp.s) Ground Black Pepper

Keto Ham And Bean Soup

No compelling reason to miss beans on a low carb diet. This Keto Ham and Bean Soup formula utilize a mystery, keto bean substitute that preferences simply like the genuine article.

Ingredients

- 1 cup (186 g) dried dark soybeans, doused to yield 2 cups beans
- 1 cup (160 g) onions, slashed
- 1 cup (101 g) slashed celery
- 4 cloves (4 cloves) Minced Garlic
- 1 Tbsp. (1 Tbsp.) Dried Oregano
- .5 to 1 Tbsp. salt
- 1 Tbsp. (1 Tbsp.) Cajun Seasoning
- 1 Tbsp. (1 Tbsp.) Liquid Smoke
- 2 Tbsp.s (2 Tbsp.s) Tony Chachere's universally handy flavoring
- 1 Tbsp. (1 Tbsp.) Louisiana Hot sauce
- 1 (1) substantial ham bone or 2 smoked ham sells
- 2 cups (280 g) slashed ham

- 2 cups (16.91 floz) Water

Simple Mango Cardamom Pannacotta

Low Carb Panna Cotta sets up rapidly and is a reviving summer dessert. Delicious, rich panna cotta joined with sweet mango.

Ingredients

- 1 tablespoon (1 tablespoon) unflavored gelatin
- 2 cups (488 g) Fairlife entire milk, (separated)
- 1 cup (165 g) mango
- 1 cup (238 g) Heavy Whipping Cream
- 1/2 cup (91 g) Swerve, or other sugar
- 1 Tbsp. (1 Tbsp.) Ground Cardamom

Smooth SHRIMP SCAMPI

Simple Low Carb Keto Creamy Shrimp Scampi from your moment pot or weight cooker, this one cooks quick! Put it over some low carb noodles for a snappy supper.

Ingredients

- 2 tablespoons Butter
- 1 pound Shrimp, solidified
- 4 cloves Garlic, minced
- 1/4-1/2 Tbsp.s Red Pepper Flakes
- 1/2 Tbsp.s Smoked Paprika
- 2 cups Carbanada low carb pasta, (uncooked)

- 1 cup Chicken Broth

- 1/2 cup Half and Half

- 1/2 cup Parmesan Cheese

- Salt, to taste

- Ground Black Pepper, to taste

Moment POT SPAGHETTI SQUASH

When you make Spaghetti squash in the Instant pot, you will never make it another way. Eight minutes under tension, without cutting the squash, and you have the ideal low carb or veggie lover side dish.

Ingredients

- 1 Large Spaghetti Squash
- 1.5 cups Water, for the Instant Pot

Tomato Eggplant Soup

This is such an extraordinary vegan Tomato Eggplant Soup formula! Empty everything into your Instant Pot, and you'll have a magnificent Mediterranean soup for supper in less than 30 minutes.

Ingredients

- 3 tablespoons Oil

- 2 tablespoons Minced Garlic

- 4 cups Eggplant, slashed

- 2 cups Tomatoes, slashed, or 1 14.5 ounce canned tomatoes, depleted

- 1 cup Onion, slashed
- 1 cup ringer pepper, cleaved
- 1/2 cup Water
- 1 Tbsp. salt
- 1 Tbsp. Ground Black Pepper

Moment Pot Sauerkraut Soup Recipe

Utilize your Instant Pot to make this flavorful, low-carb Sauerkraut Soup formula! It's a simple dump and cooks formula that cooks in a short time.

Ingredients

- 1 cup dried cannellini beans, drenched medium-term and depleted
- 14 oz smoked frankfurters, cut down the middle longwise, and afterward cut into 1-inch pieces
- 1 cup sauerkraut with brackish water
- 3 Bay Leaves
- 1 cup onions, slashed
- 1 tablespoon Minced Garlic
- 1 Tbsp. Salt
- 1 Tbsp. Ground Black Pepper
- 4 cups Water

Chicken And Mushrooms Recipe

If you need to make a Chicken and Mushrooms Recipe, however, would prefer not to utilize canned soup, have I got only the thing for you! It's Keto and Instant Pot also!

Ingredients

- 2 tablespoons (2 tablespoons) Butter
- 1 cup (160 g) Sliced Onions
- 6 (6) Garlic Cloves, cut slender
- 1 cup (186 g) Mushrooms, cut into quarters
- 1 lb (453.59 g) Boneless Skinless Chicken Thighs
- 4 cups (120 g) infant spinach
- 2 tablespoons (2 tablespoons) Water
- 1 Tbsp.ful of Dried Thyme, or 3-4 sprigs crisp thyme
- 1 Tbsp. (1 Tbsp.) Salt
- 1 Tbsp.ful of Ground Black Pepper
- For Finishing
- 1/2 cup (119 g) Heavy Whipping Cream
- 1 tablespoon (1 tablespoon) lemon juice

Keto Shrimp Scampi

8 minutes from beginning to end to make this air fryer keto low carb shrimp scampi. So easy to make, so heavenly, you will have a hard time believing it.

Ingredients

- 4 tablespoons (4 tablespoons) Butter
- 1 tablespoon (1 tablespoon) lemon juice
- 1 tablespoon (1 tablespoon) Minced Garlic
- 2 Tbsp.s (2 Tbsp.s) Red Pepper Flakes
- 1 tablespoon (1 tablespoon) hacked chives, or 1 Tbsp. dried chives
- 1 tablespoon (1 tablespoon) hacked crisp basil, or 1 Tbsp. dried basil
- 2 tablespoons of Chicken Stock, (or white wine)
- 1 lb (453.59 g) defrosted shrimp, (21-25 check)

Essential Indian Curry Recipe | Pressure Cooker Curry Recipe

This Basic Indian Curry is a tasty customary Indian curry formula made in the Instant Pot! This curry formula is low-carb and stuffed with Indian flavor.

Ingredients

- 1 pound (453.59 g) Boneless Pork Shoulder, diced into 2 inch 3D squares
- 1.5 cups (240 g) onions, hacked
- 1 cup (242 g) Canned Tomatoes, undrained
- 1 tablespoon (1 tablespoon) Minced Garlic
- 1 tablespoon minced ginger
- 2 Tbsp.s (2 Tbsp.s) Garam Masala, separated
- 1 Tbsp. (1 Tbsp.) Salt

- 1 Tbsp. (1 Tbsp.) Turmeric
- 1/4-1 Tbsp. (0.25 Tbsp.) Cayenne
- 2 tablespoons (2 tablespoons) Water

Chicken Tikka Masala

Make simple, real Chicken Tikka Masala comfortable in your Instant Pot or weight cooker! It's by a wide margin the simplest method to make Chicken Tikka Masala.

Ingredients

Marinate the chicken

- 1 ½ pound (680.39 g) Boneless Skinless Chicken Thighs, (bosom or thighs), cut into enormous pieces
- ½ cups (100 g) Greek Yogurt
- 4 cloves (4 cloves) Garlic, minced
- 2 Tbsp.s (2 Tbsp.s) minced ginger, minced
- ½ Tbsp. (0.5 Tbsp.) Turmeric
- ¼ Tbsp. (0.25 Tbsp.) Cayenne
- ½ Tbsp. (0.5 Tbsp.s) Smoked Paprika, for shading and a somewhat smoky taste
- 1 Tbsp. (1 Tbsp.) Salt
- 1 Tbsp. (1 Tbsp.) Garam Masala
- 1/2 Tbsp. (0.5 Tbsp.s) Ground Cumin
- 1 Tbsp. (1 Tbsp.) Liquid Smoke, (overlook if inaccessible)

Simple Traditional Keto Chaffle

Ingredients

- 1 Egg
- 1/2 cup Shredded Cheddar Cheese

Directions

- Preheat mini waffle creator.
- In a cucp, whisk the egg until beaten.
- Add destroyed cheddar and mix to consolidate.
- When the waffle creator is warmed, cautiously pour 1/2 of the hitter in the waffle producer and close the top. Permit to cook for 3-5 minutes.
- Carefully expel from the waffle producer and put in a safe spot for 2-3 minutes to fresh up.
- Repeat guidelines again for the second chaffle.

Keto Strawberry Shortcake Chaffle

Ingredients

- 1 Egg
- 1 tbsp Heavy Whipping Cream
- 1 tsp Coconut Flour
- 2 tbsp Lakanto Golden Sweetener (Use butter together for 20% off)
- 1/2 tsp Cake Batter Extract
- 1/4 tsp Baking powder

Keto Pumpkin Cheesecake Chaffle

Ingredients

PUMPKIN CHAFFLE

- 1 Egg
- 1/2 cup Mozzarella Cheese
- 1 1/2 tbsp Pumpkin Puree (100% pumpkin)
- 1 tbsp Almond Flour
- 1 tbsp Lakanto Golden Sweetener, or decision of sugar
- 2 tsp Heavy Cream
- 1 tsp Cream Cheese, relaxed
- 1/2 tsp Pumpkin Spice
- 1/2 tsp Baking Powder
- 1/2 tsp Vanilla
- 1 tsp Choczero Maple Syrup or 1/8 tsp Maple Extract

Tasty Keto Pizza Chaffle Recipe

Ingredients

CHAFFLE CRUST

- 1 Egg
- 1/2 cup Mozzarella Cheese
- 1 tsp Coconut Flour
- 1/4 tsp Baking Powder
- 1/8 tsp Garlic Powder

- 1/8 tsp Italian Seasoning
- Pinch of Salt

Pizza Topping

- 1 tbsp Rao's Marinara Sauce
- 1/2 cup Mozzarella Cheese
- 3 Pepperoni's, cut into four
- Shredded Parmesan Cheese, discretionary
- Parsley, discretionary

Best Oreo Keto Chaffles

Ingredients

CHOCOLATE CHAFFLE

- 1 Egg
- 1 1/2 tbsp Unsweetened Cocoa
- 2 tbsp Lakanto Monkfruit, or decision of sugar
- 1 tbsp Heavy Cream
- 1 tsp Coconut Flour
- 1/2 tsp Baking Powder
- 1/2 tsp Vanilla

FILLING

- Whipped Cream (interchange icing formula in notes beneath)

Guidelines

- Preheat mini waffle producer.

- In a small bowl, join all chaffle ingredients.
- Pour a portion of the chaffle blend into the focal point of the waffle iron. Permit to cook for 3-5 minutes.

Keto Peanut Butter Cup Chaffle

Ingredients

CHAFFLE

- 1 Egg
- 1 tbsp Heavy Cream
- 1 tbsp Unsweetened Cocoa
- 1 tbsp Lakanto Powdered Sweetener
- 1 tsp Coconut Flour
- 1/2 tsp Vanilla Extract
- 1/2 Cake Batter Flavor (we utilize this)
- 1/4 tsp Baking Powder

Nutty spread FILLING

- 3 tbsp All regular Peanut Butter
- 2 tsp Lakanto Powdered Sweetener
- 2 tbsp Heavy Cream

Keto Snickerdoodle Chaffle

Ingredients

- 1 Egg
- 1/2 cup Mozzarella Cheese

- 2 tbsp Almond Flour
- 1 tbsp Lakanto Golden Sweetener
- 1/2 tsp Vanilla Extract
- 1/4 tsp Cinnamon
- 1/2 tsp Baking Powder
- 1/4 tsp Cream of tartar, discretionary

Covering

- 1 tbsp Butter
- 2 tbsp Lakanto Classic Sweetener
- 1/2 tsp Cinnamon

Guidelines

- Preheat your mini waffle producer.
- In a little bowl, join all chaffle ingredients.
- Pour a portion of the chaffle blend on to the focal point of the waffle iron. Permit to cook for 3-5 minutes.
- Carefully expel and rehash for the second chaffle. Permit chaffles to cool so they fresh.
- In a little bowl, consolidate sugar and cinnamon for covering.
- Melt spread in a little microwave-safe bowl and brush the chaffles with the margarine.
- Sprinkle sugar and cinnamon blend on the two sides of the chaffles once they're brushed with margarine.

White Bread Keto Chaffle | Wonder Bread Chaffle

Ingredients

- 1 Egg
- 3 tbsp Almond Flour
- 1 tbsp Mayonnaise
- 1/4 tsp Baking Powder
- 1 tsp Water

Guidelines

- Preheat mini waffle producer.
- In a cup, whisk the egg until beaten.
- Add almond flour, mayonnaise, heating powder, and water.
- When the waffle producer is warmed, cautiously pour 1/2 of the hitter in the waffle creator and close the top. Permit to cook for 3-5 minutes.
- Carefully expel from the waffle creator and put in a safe spot for 2-3 minutes to fresh up.
- Repeat directions again for the second chaffle.

Best Oreo Keto Chaffles

Ingredients

CHOCOLATE CHAFFLE

- 1 Egg
- 1 1/2 tbsp Unsweetened Cocoa

- 2 tbsp Lakanto Monkfruit, or decision of sugar
- 1 tbsp Heavy Cream
- 1 tsp Coconut Flour
- 1/2 tsp Baking Powder
- 1/2 tsp Vanilla

FILLING

- Whipped Cream (exchange icing formula in notes beneath)

Guidelines

- Preheat mini waffle producer.
- In a small bowl, join all chaffle ingredients.
- Pour a portion of the chaffle blend into the focal point of the waffle iron. Permit to cook for 3-5 minutes.

Keto Chocolate Chip Chaffle Keto Recipe

Ingredients

- 1 egg
- 1 tbsp substantial whipping cream
- 1/2 tsp coconut flour
- 1 3/4 tsp Lakanto monk fruit brilliant can utilize pretty much to change the sweetness
- 1/4 tsp preparing powder
- pinch of salt
- 1 tbsp Lily's Chocolate Chips

Directions

1. Turn on the waffle creator with the goal that it warms up.
2. In a little bowl, join all ingredients with the exception of the chocolate chips and mix well until consolidated.
3. Grease waffle producer, at that point, pour half of the hitter onto the base plate of the waffle creator.
4. Cook it for 5 minutes or until the chocolate chip chaffle pastry is brilliant dark colored at that point expel from waffle creator with a fork, being mindful so as not to burn your fingers.

Keto Strawberry Cheesecake Shake

Ingredients

- 1 cup Almond Milk, unsweetened
- 2oz Cream cheddar
- 1/2 cup Strawberries
- 2 tbsp Heavy cream
- 1 tbsp Lakanto monk fruit, or decision of sugar
- 1/2 tsp Vanilla
- 1 tbsp ChocZero Strawberry Syrup, discretionary

Directions

1. Add every one of the ingredients into a blender and mix until smooth. Include ice-blocks varying. Appreciate!

Keto Taco Chaffle Recipe (Crispy Taco Shells)

Ingredients

- 1 egg white

- 1/4 cup Monterey jack cheddar, destroyed (stuffed firmly)
- 1/4 cup sharp cheddar, destroyed (stuffed firmly)
- 3/4 tsp water
- 1 tsp coconut flour
- 1/4 tsp preparing powder
- 1/8 tsp stew powder
- pinch of salt

Directions

1. Plug the Dash Mini Waffle Maker in the divider and oil delicately once it is hot.
2. Combine the entirety of the ingredients in a bowl and mix to consolidate.
3. Spoon out 1/2 of the player on the waffle creator and close top. Set a clock for 4 minutes and don't lift the cover until the cooking time is finished. In the event that you do, it will resemble the taco chaffle shell isn't set up appropriately. However it will. You need to let it cook the whole 4 minutes before lifting the cover.

Maple Pumpkin Keto Waffle Recipe (Chaffle)

Ingredients

- 2 eggs
- 3/4 tsp heating powder
- 2 tsp pumpkin puree (100% pumpkin)
- 3/4 tsp pumpkin pie zest

- 4 tsp substantial whipping cream
- 2 tsp Lakanto Sugar-Free Maple Syrup
- 1 tsp coconut flour
- 1/2 cup mozzarella cheddar, destroyed
- 1/2 tsp vanilla
- pinch of salt

Guidelines

1. Turn on a waffle or chaffle producer. I utilize the Dash Mini Waffle Maker.
2. In a little bowl, join all ingredients.
3. Cover the scramble mini waffle producer with 1/4 of the player and cook for 3-4 minutes.
4. Repeat 3 additional occasions until you have made 4 Maple Syrup Pumpkin Keto Waffles (Chaffles).
5. Serve with without sugar maple syrup or keto frozen yogurt.

Keto Chaffle Breakfast Sandwich

Ingredients
- 1 egg
- 1/2 cup Monterey Jack Cheese
- 1 tablespoon almond flour
- 2 tablespoons spread

Directions

1. In a little bowl, blend the egg, almond flour, and Monterey Jack Cheese.

2. Pour a portion of the hitter into your mini waffle creator and cook for 3-4 minutes. At that point, cook the remainder of the player to make a second chaffle.

3. In a little container, dissolve 2 tablespoons of spread. Include the chaffles and cook each side for 2 minutes. Pushing down while they are cooking gently on the highest point of them, so they are fresh up better.

4. Remove from the container and let sit for 2 minutes.

Mini Keto Pizza Recipe

Ingredients

- 1/2 cup Shredded Mozzarella cheddar
- 1 tablespoon almond flour
- 1/2 tsp heating powder
- 1 egg
- 1/4 tsp garlic powder
- 1/4 tsp basil
- 2 tablespoons low carb pasta sauce
- 2 tablespoons mozzarella cheddar

Guidelines

1. While the waffle producer is warming up, in a bowl blend mozzarella cheddar, preparing powder, garlic, premise, egg, and almond flour.
2. Pour 1/2 the blend into your mini waffle producer.
3. Cook it for 3-5 min. until your pizza waffle is totally cooked. On the off chance that you check it and the waffle adheres to the waffle creator, let it cook for one more moment or two.

Sugar-Free Vanilla Buttercream Frosting

Ingredients

- 1 cup margarine room temperature
- 1.5 cups swerve confectioner
- 2 tbsp Heavy Whipping Cream
- 1 tsp vanilla concentrate

Guidelines

1. Place your margarine and swerve in the bowl of your blender. Combine them on low speed until the sugar is joined.
2. Mix in the substantial cream and the vanilla concentrate.
3. Turn the blender up to medium-fast and keep blending for 6-8 minutes until light and feathery.

Keto Blueberry Chaffle

This scrumptious keto blueberry waffles are, in fact, called a Keto Chaffle! What's more, a kid is it delish! Consummately sweet, with succulent blueberries, these blueberry keto chaffles taste extraordinary and are low carb and keto well disposed.

Ingredients

- 1 cup of mozzarella cheddar
- 2 tablespoons almond flour
- 1 tsp preparing powder
- 2 eggs
- 1 tsp cinnamon
- 2 tsp of Swerve
- 3 tablespoon blueberries

Directions

1. Heat up your Dash mini waffle creator.
2. In a blending bowl include the mozzarella cheddar, almond flour, preparing powder, eggs, cinnamon, swerve, and blueberries. Blend well, so every one of the ingredients is combined.
3. Spray your mini waffle creator with non-stick cooking splash.
4. Add shortly less than 1/4 a cup of blueberry keto waffle hitter.

Bacon Cheddar Chaffles Recipe

- 1 egg
- 1.2 cup cheddar
- Bacon bits to taste
- Mix and cook until fresh.

Bacon Jalapeno Chaffles Recipe

1. 1/2 cup destroyed swiss/gruyere mix
2. 1 egg
3. 2 tablespoons cooked bacon pieces
4. 1 tablespoon diced crisp jalapenos
5. Cook until fresh. Works incredibly as a bun to a cheeseburger.

Keto Cauliflower Chaffles Recipe

You can make the most delightful keto cauliflower chaffle formula with only a bunch of ingredients and a couple of moments! This formula will be your new top choice!

Ingredients

- 1 cup riced cauliflower
- 1/4 Tbsp. Garlic Powder
- 1/4 Tbsp. Ground Black Pepper
- 1/2 Tbsp. Italian Seasoning
- 1/4 Tbsp. salt
- 1/2 cup destroyed mozzarella cheddar or destroyed Mexican mix cheddar
- 1 Egg
- 1/2 cup destroyed parmesan cheddar

Sandwich Bread Chaffles Recipe

- 1 egg

- 2 tablespoon almond flour
- 1 tablespoon mayo
- 1/8 Tbsp. heating powder
- 1 Tbsp. water
- Sweetener and garlic powder (discretionary)
- Makes 2 chaffles, and you can undoubtedly slice them down the middle for a bun.

Sweet Chaffles Recipes

To make chaffles sweet, the conceivable outcomes are inestimable! You can just utilize the base formula and include some Keto-accommodating sugars.

In the event that you need to include some sweet seasoning after, you can sprinkle a wide range of Keto-accommodating magnificence on top. I like to utilize this Lakanto Maple Syrup. Something else, on the off chance that you need more than that, you can use the recipes beneath!

Chocolate Brownie Chaffles

- Making the Keto Chocolate Brownies Batter.
- Stir and pour in the mini waffle producer.
- You can see the entire formula and a video here for how to make chocolate chaffles
- Cook 5-7 minutes until firm. – TwoSleevers

Mint Chocolate Broffle (Brownie Waffle)

- Use this keto brownie formula.
- Add hacked walnuts, and each broffle (brownie waffle) utilized 3 tablespoons of player for 7 min.
- The formula for the buttercream depends on Urvashi's maple walnut buttercream formula, just with mint rather than maple separate.

Lemon Pound Cake Chaffles

Numerous individuals are cutting my lemon pound cake formula by 1/4 and making Cake Chaffles out of them.

Crusty fruit-filled treat CHAFFLES

- 1.2 cup mozzarella cheddar
- 1 egg
- Add the mozzarella to the waffle producer.
- Put the egg on top.
- Sprinkle on crusty fruit-filled treat zest and 5 sugar-free chocolate chips.
- Serve with margarine on top.

Cream Cheese Carrot Cake Chaffles

- 2 tablespoons cream cheddar or a blend of 1 tablespoon cream cheddar and 2 tablespoons destroyed mozzarella cheddar
- 1/2 pat of margarine
- 1 tablespoon finely destroyed carrot

- 1 tablespoon of sugar of your decision. I utilized Splenda.
- 1 tablespoon almond flour
- 1 Tbsp. pumpkin pie zest
- 1/2 Tbsp. vanilla
- 1/2 Tbsp. heating powder
- 1 egg
- OPTIONAL

I included 6 raisins, 1 tablespoon of destroyed coconut, and 1/2 tablespoon of pecans to the blender ingredients.

Cream Cheese Frosting

- 1 tablespoon cream cheddar
- 1 pat spread
- 1 Tbsp. sugar of decision. I utilized Cinnamon Brown Sugar without sugar syrup.
- Heat up, waffle creator. I utilized a mini Dash. I oiled with a silicon brush dunked in coconut oil.
- Microwave cream cheddar, mozzarella, and spread for 15 seconds to liquefy the cheeses to make consolidating simpler. I did this in an enchantment slug cup to mix.
- Add the remainder of the chaffle ingredients to the blender cup and mix until smooth and consolidated.
- Add a player to a waffle creator. For the Dash, I included 2 stacking tablespoons, and it made 3 chaffles.

- While making the chaffle, heat up the spread and cream cheddar for the icing. Blend until smooth, and consolidate your sugar. Sprinkle over chaffles as wanted.

Cinnamon Chaffles

- 1/2 cup mozzarella
- 1 egg
- 1 tbsp vanilla concentrate
- 1/2 tsp preparing powder
- 1 tbsp almond flour
- Sprinkle of cinnamon
- Mix together and cook until chaffles are firm.

Cinnamon Swirl Chaffles

- CHAFFLE:
- 1 oz cream cheddar, mollified
- 1 huge egg, beaten
- 1 tsp vanilla concentrate
- 1 tbsp almond flour, superfine
- 1 tbsp Splenda
- 1 tsp cinnamon
- ICING:
- 1 oz cream cheddar, mollified
- 1 tbsp. spread, unsalted

- 1 tbsp Splenda
- 1/2 tsp vanilla

Cinnamon Drizzle:

- 1/2 tbsp spread
- 1 tbsp Splenda
- 1 tsp cinnamon
- Heat up waffle creator, and I brushed on coconut oil on my DASH.
- Stir up the chaffle ingredients until smooth.
- Utilize a spoon to include 2 piling tbsp of the player to the waffle iron. It will make 3 little waffles.
- Cook to your ideal waffle freshness. I did 4 min. They resembled a delicate waffle.
- Cool on a rack.
- Mix the icing and cinnamon shower in little dishes. Warmth in the microwave for 10 secs to find a workable pace consistency. Whirl on cooled waffles.

Greek Marinated Feta And Olives

Ingredients

- 1 cup olive oil
- 1/4 Tbsp. oregano
- 1/4 Tbsp. thyme
- 1/2 Tbsp. dried rosemary
- 1 cup kalamata olives

- 1 cup of green olives
- 1/2 pound feta

Directions

- In a little pot heat, the oil, oregano, thyme, rosemary together over medium warmth for 5 minutes to imbue the oil with the herbs.
- Set the oil to the side and enable it to cool for 15 minutes.
- Cut the feta into 1/2 inch 3D shapes.

Air Fryer Peanut Chicken

Not many things state "Thai food" like Peanut Chicken. This Peanut Chicken formula takes the dish to an unheard-of level and is effectively made in your air fryer!

Ingredients

- 1 pound Bone-in Skin-on Chicken Thighs
- For the Sauce
- 1/4 cup Creamy Peanut Butter
- 1 tablespoon Sriracha Sauce, (modify for your zest needs)
- 1 tablespoon Soy Sauce
- 2 tablespoons sweet chili sauce
- 2 tablespoons lime juice
- 1 Tbsp. Minced Garlic
- 1 Tbsp. minced ginger
- 1/2 Tbsp. salt, to taste
- 1/2 cup high temp water

Green Beans With Bacon

Right now, Pot Green Beans with Bacon formula is a fast, low carb, and nutritious dish that can be eaten either as a side dish or as a low carb dinner. Just beans, bacon, and a couple of seasonings make this a quick and simple dish.

Ingredients

- 1 cup (160 g) onion, diced
- 5 cuts (5 cuts) Bacon, diced
- 6 cups (660 g) green beans, cut in

Keto Buffalo Chicken Casserole

This Buffalo Chicken Casserole is as flavorful filling dish with the perfect measure of kick! It's the ideal weeknight supper that requires little exertion to make.

Ingredients

- 4 cups rotisserie chicken, destroyed
- 1/2 cup Onion, slashed
- 1/4 cup Cream
- 1/4 cup hot wing sauce
- 1/4 cup blue cheddar, disintegrated
- 2 ounces Cream Cheese, diced
- pepper
- 1/4 cup Green Onions, slashed

German Red Cabbage

Appreciate this customary German Red Cabbage formula made in a non-conventional way! Make this wonderfully prepared side dish directly in your Instant Pot!

Ingredients

- 6 cups red cabbage, cleaved
- 3 Granny Smith Apples, little, cut 1 inch thick
- 2 tablespoons liquefied margarine, or oil
- 1/3 cup Apple Cider Vinegar
- 2-3 tablespoons Sugar
- 1 Tbsp. salt
- 1/2 Tbsp. Ground Black Pepper
- 1/4 Tbsp. Ground Cloves
- 2 sound leaves

Maple Pecan Bars With Sea Salt

Ingredients

For the Crust

- Non-Stick Spray
- 1/3 cup Butter, mellowed
- 1/4 cup Brown Sugar, immovably stuffed
- 1 cup All-Purpose Flour
- 1/4 Kosher tea Salt

For the Filling

- 4 TBS Butter (1/2 stick), diced
- 1/2 cup Brown Sugar
- 1/4 cup Pure Maple Syrup
- 1/4 cup Whole Milk
- 1/4 tea Vanilla concentrate

Moment Pot Vegetarian Chili

Ingredients

- 1 cup Onion, cleaved
- 1 cup Canned Fire Roasted Tomatoes
- 1.5 tablespoons Minced Garlic
- 3 corn tortillas
- 1 tablespoon Chipotle Chile in Adobo Sauce, cleaved
- 1 tablespoon Mexican Red Chili Powder, (not cayenne)
- 2 Tbsp.s Ground Cumin
- 2 Tbsp.s salt
- 1 Tbsp. Dried Oregano
- 1 cup Water
- 1/2 cup dried pinto beans, doused medium-term or for 1 hour in heated water
- 1/2 cup dried dark beans, splashed medium-term or for 1 hour in high temp water
- 2 cups corn, new or defrosted solidified corn

- 2 cups zucchini, hacked

Keto Almendrados Cookies | Spanish Almond Keto Cookies

Ingredients

- 1.5 cups Superfine Almond Flour
- 1/2 cup Swerve
- 1 huge Egg
- 1 Tbsp. Lemon Extract
- 1 tablespoon lemon get-up-and-go
- 24 whitened almonds

Directions

1. In a medium bowl, beat egg. Include almond flour, swerve and lemon and combine to make a strong mixture. Cover and refrigerate for 1-2 hours.
2. Preheat stove to 350 degrees. Line a heating sheet with material paper.
3. Pinching off bits of batter about the size of a pecan, fold them into balls.

Keto Taco

Prep. time: 11 minutes/Cook time: 20 minutes/Serves 3

Need to begin the day surprising? Morning keto is such an astounding beginning to a delightful day. Light and superb with a lot of splendid hues and feelings.

8 oz. Mozzarella cheddar, destroyed; 6 Eggs, enormous 2 tbsp. Margarine

3 Bacon stripes ½ Avocado 1 oz. Cheddar, destroyed Pepper and salt to taste

Keto Omelet With Goat Cheese And Spinach

Prep. time: 5 minutes

3 Large eggs 1 Medium green onion 1 oz. Goat cheddar ¼ Onion

2 tbsp. Margarine 2 cups Spinach 2 tbsp. Substantial cream Salt and pepper to taste

Chicken And Cheese Quesadilla

Prep. time: 10 minutes/Serves 4

For capsules: 6 Eggs 4 oz. Coconut flour 6 oz. Substantial cream ½ tsp. Thickener Pink salt and pepper 1 tbsp. Olive oil for fricasseeing

For the quesadilla: 4 oz. Cheddar destroyed 8 oz. Chicken bosom cooked and destroyed 1 tbsp. Parsley, cleaved (discretionary)

Gluten Free Sports Nutrition Basics

At the point when you're a competitor, it's imperative to get a decent assortment of protein, sugars, and sound fats for the duration of the day. Evading gluten implies picking gluten-free nourishments and wiping out wheat, grain, and rye items from your eating routine to keep away from aggravation, swelling, stomach torment, cramps, looseness of the bowels, exhaustion, lack of healthy sustenance, iron deficiency, and blockage.

Protein Needs

The American College of Sports Medicine and the Academy of Nutrition and Dietetics prescribe athletes eat 0.5 to 0.8 grams of protein per pound of their body weight day by day, and 15 to 20 percent of their complete calories from protein.

Pick a lot of protein-rich nourishments, for example,

- Lean meats, poultry, fish, and fish
- Eggs
- Low-fat dairy nourishments or dairy substitutes
- Tofu or other soy items
- Legumes
- Nuts, seeds, and nut margarines

Carb Requirements

Carbs are essential for athletes since this macronutrient is a competitor's primary vitality source. Athletes get 50 to 60 percent of their calories from carbs, or 2.7 to 4.6 grams of carbs per pound of body weight day by day. Pick sound, gluten-free carbs, for example,

- Gluten-free oats, oats, and oats (must indicate gluten-free)
- Rice
- Quinoa
- Fruits
- Starchy vegetables like potatoes, yams, peas, corn, and vegetables

Fat Recommendations

Dietary fat should make up around 20 to 30 percent of a competitor's calorie consumption. Pick sound fats, for example,

- Nuts and seeds
- Nut margarines
- Plant-based oils
- Avocadoes
- Olives

Gluten Free Recipes for Athletes

Gluten Free Recipes For Athletes

The accompanying gluten-free recipes make certain to be a hit with athletes, regardless of whether utilized before working out for a snappy increase in vitality or as a post-practice recuperation feast or bite.

Almond Blast Protein Shake

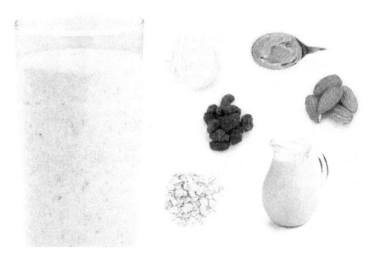

This shake assists athletes with devouring protein, which is basic for muscle improvement.

Fixings

- 2 scoops of gluten-free vanilla-seasoned protein powder
- 1.5 cups of low-fat milk, soy milk, or almond milk
- ½ cup of gluten-free oats
- ½ cup of raisins

- 12 fragmented almonds

- 1 tablespoon of nutty spread

Bearings

Mix all fixings together in blender and serve chilled.

Chocolate Peanut Butter Protein Balls

Anoth er protein-rich formula, these protein balls make an incredible pre- or post-exercise nibble.

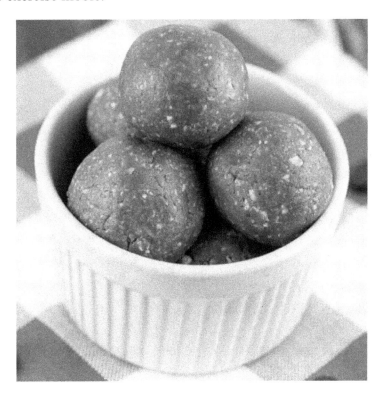

Fixings

- 1 cup of gluten-free moved oats

- 1/2 cup of characteristic nutty spread
- 1/3 cup of nectar
- 2 tablespoons of flax seeds
- 2 tablespoons of chia seeds
- 1 tablespoon of gluten-free chocolate protein powder

Bearings

1. Stir all fixings together in a bowl.
2. Cover the bowl with cling wrap.
3. Refrigerate blend for 30 minutes.
4. Scoop chilled blend into balls and serve.

Tomato Spinach Omelet

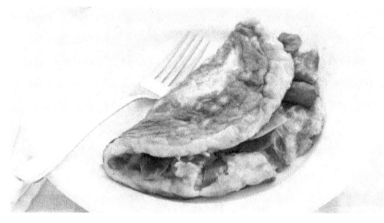

With sound protein and nutrient-thick veggies, this formula is an extraordinary method to begin the day.

Fixings

- 4 enormous eggs

- 1/2 cup broiler cooked tomatoes

- 1 cup infant spinach leaves

- 1/2 cup feta cheddar

- 1 tablespoon olive oil

Headings

1. Saute the spinach and tomatoes in the olive oil over medium-low warmth for a few minutes.

2. Pour the beaten eggs into the skillet and gradually shake to circulate equitably all through.

3. After around two minutes, slacken the omelet blend from the base of the container to forestall staying.

4. Sprinkle the feta cheddar over the omelet.

5. Fold the omelet with the cheddar in the center and cook until it is brilliant darker.

6. Flip the omelet and cook for one increasingly minute.

7. Serve with gluten-free toast and orange cuts, whenever wanted.

Quinoa And Asparagus Chicken Salad

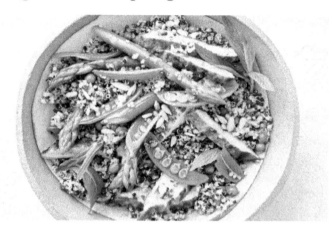

This formula is an extraordinary wellspring of gluten-free complex carbs and protein.

Fixings

- 1/2 cup uncooked quinoa
- 2 ounces chicken bosom
- 1/2 cup sun-dried tomatoes
- 10-ounces asparagus
- 1/2 cup feta cheddar
- 1 tablespoon olive oil
- Salt and pepper

Headings

1. Cook the quinoa as guided and add it to an enormous bowl.
2. Steam the asparagus for around 5 minutes and cut it into little pieces.

3.   Add the asparagus, tomatoes, feta cheddar, and chicken bosom to bowl with the quinoa.

4.   Add the olive oil, salt, and pepper.

5.   Mix all fixings and appreciate!

Turkey Chili

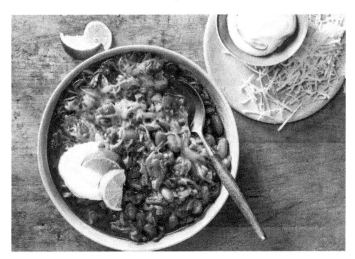

Lean protein, complex carbs, and bunches of flavor makes this a thought formula for athletes.

Fixings

- 2 cups water
- 1 pound ground turkey
- 1 jar of diced tomatoes
- 1 jar of kidney beans
- 1 slashed onion
- 1 1/2 Tbsp.s olive oil

- 1 tablespoon minced garlic
- 2 tablespoons bean stew powder
- 1/2 Tbsp. oregano
- 1/2 Tbsp. ground cumin
- 1/2 Tbsp. paprika
- Salt and pepper to taste

Headings

1. Cook the turkey and olive oil in a pot over medium warmth until darker.
2. Add the onions and cook until delicate.
3. Add the rest of the fixings and heat the blend to the point of boiling.
4. Reduce the warmth to low and stew for about 30 minutes.

Anti-Aging Recipes

Edamame With Ground Bonito And Seaweed

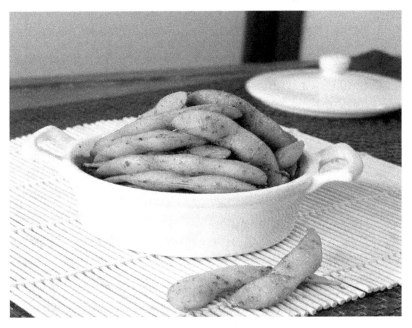

Prep Time: 5 Minutes/ Cook Time: 6 Minutes/ Total Time: 11 Minutes/

Category: Snack/ Cuisine: Vegetarian

Fixings

- 1 pound edamame (new or solidified)
- 1/4 nori sheet
- 2 tablespoons bonito chips
- 1/2 Tbsp. salt

Directions

1. Follow bearings on edamame bundle on how to cook them (I lean toward bubbling them two or three minutes not as much as what the headings state, as it makes them less soft). Channel them and let them dry for 2-3 minutes.

2. Break the nori and add it to an espresso/flavor processor alongside the bonito pieces and the salt. Granulate the blend until it nearly transforms into a powder.

3. Put the edamame in a blending bowl and sprinkle the powdered blend over them. Hurl a couple of times and serve.

Korean Pickles

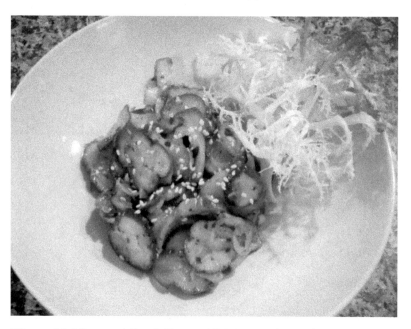

Prep Time: 10 Minutes/ Cook Time: 15 Minutes/ Total Time: 25 Minutes/
Category: Condiment/ Cuisine: Korean

Fixings

- 2 cups daikon (stripped and julienned (cut into little strips))
- 1 medium carrot (stripped and julienned)
- 1 shallot (finely hacked)
- 2 tablespoons water
- 3 tablespoons rice vinegar
- 2 Tbsp.s tobanjan (Korean stew glue)
- 2 Tbsp.s sesame oil
- 1 Tbsp. granulated sugar
- 2 Tbsp.s salt (in addition to included 1/2 Tbsp.)
- 1 tablespoon sesame seeds

Directions

1. Put the daikon, carrots and shallot in a medium size blending bowl and include 2 tsp salt. Rapidly blend in with your hands and leave for 10 minutes, to mollify the veggies.

2. In a different little bowl, blend water, rice vinegar and tobanjan. Mix until tobanjan has weakened and include sugar, 1/2 tsp salt, and sesame oil. Mix well until sugar and salt have dissolved.

3. Rinse the vegetable, channel and press out overabundance water. Return the vegetable in the blending bowl and pour the tobanjan blend over.

4. Add sesame seeds and utilizing chopsticks or a spoon, blend until veggies are all around covered. Serve or let pickle for as long as 3 days.

Nourishment

- Calories: 233

- Saturated Fat: 2

Pan Fried Food Beef With Spicy Hoisin Sauce

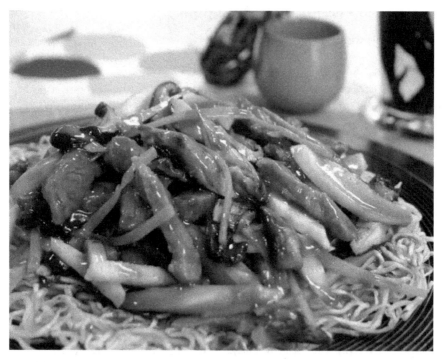

Make this hot, valid Szechuan hoisin pan sear hamburger formula in under 20 minutes!

Prep Time: 10 Minutes/ Cook Time: 6 Minutes/ Total Time: 16 Minutes/
Yield: 2 People 1x/ Category: Main/ Cuisine: Chinese

Fixings

- 1/2 pound lean meat (meagerly cut scaled down)

- 1 red chime pepper (center and seeded, cut into meager strips (julienne))
- 4 scallions (generally cleaved)
- 1 tablespoon vegetable oil
- 2 cloves garlic (finely cleaved)
- 2 Thai bean stews (finely slashed)
- 2 tablespoons hoisin sauce
- 1 Tbsp. white miso glue
- For the marinade:
- 1 tablespoon dull soy
- 1 tablespoon soy sauce
- 1 tablespoon shaoxing wine or dry sherry
- 1 tablespoon corn starch

Directions

1. Put all the element for the marinade in a bowl with the meat. Blend well and put in a safe spot for 30 minutes.
2. In a medium size container over high warmth, include oil, garlic and chiles and cook for 1 moment.
3. Add meat and cook for 3 minutes.
4. Add pepper and scallions and cook for 2 minutes, mixing regularly.
5. Turn the warmth off, include hoisin sauce and miso glue, mix well until glue has broken up. Serve pan sear with white rice.

Notes

This Stir Fry Beef With Hoisin Sauce:

Exceptionally high in iron

High in selenium

Extremely high in nutrient B6

Extremely high in nutrient B12

Extremely high in nutrient C

High in zinc

Sauteed Kale With Mustard Sauce

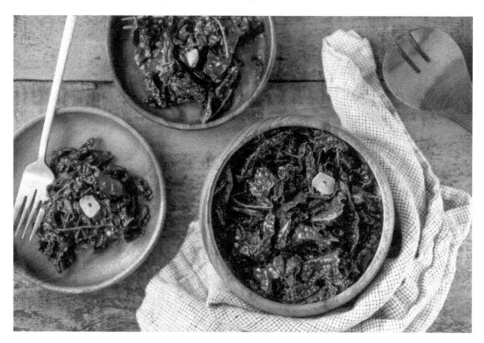

Prep Time: 5 Minutes/ Cook Time: 7 Minutes/ Total Time: 12 Minutes/
Yield: 2 1x/ Category: Side

Fixings

- 2 tablespoons additional virgin olive oil
- 1 clove garlic (minced)
- 1/4 cup white wine
- 1 pack kale (ribs expelled and finely hacked)
- 1/2 Tbsp. genuine salt
- 1/4 Tbsp. ground dark pepper
- 1 Tbsp. dijon mustard
- 1/4 cup milk

Directions

1. In a container over medium/high warmth, include olive oil and garlic. Cook for 1 moment.
2. Add white wine, mix well and cook for 1 moment.
3. Add kale, mix well and cook for 4 minutes, mixing continually.
4. Add salt and pepper, mix and cook for 1 moment.
5. Turn off the warmth, include milk and dijon mustard and rapidly mix until fluid is no more. Serve.

Sauteed Green Beans With Chilies

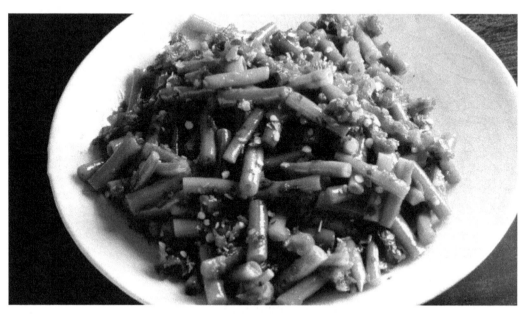

Prep Time: 10 Minutes/ Cook Time: 5 Minutes/ Total Time: 15 Minutes/

Yield: 4 1x/ Category: Side/ Cuisine: Chinese

Fixings

- 2 cloves garlic (finely hacked)

- 1 Tbsp. ginger (stripped and finely hacked)

- 1 pound green beans (washed)

- 2 tablespoons vegetable oil

- 1 Tbsp. dried red chilies (hacked)

- 1 tablespoon shellfish sauce

- 1 tablespoon soy sauce

- 1 Tbsp. sesame oil

Directions

1.   Bring a pot of salted water to bubble (not as salty as the ocean, yet enough that you can taste it).

2.   Meanwhile, flush and cut the parts of the bargains bean.

3.   When water is bubbling, whiten the green beans for 3 minutes. Channel.

4.   In a medium size container, include the vegetable oil, garlic, ginger and dried chilies. Cook for a moment and include green beans.

5.   Toss and cook for one more moment, at that point include soy sauce and clam sauce.

6.   Toss well, include sesame oil and turn the warmth off. Serve.

Nourishment

- Calories: 109
- Saturated Fat: 1

Shrimp And Celery Salad With Wasabi Mayo

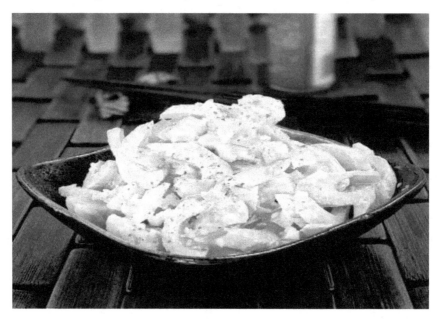

Rich, crunchy and

Prep Time: 10 Minutes/ Cook Time: 5 Minutes/ Total Time: 15 Minutes/ Yield: 4 Sides 1x/ Category: Salads/ Method: Chopping/ Cuisine: Japanese

Fixings

- 16–20 huge crude shrimps, deveined and stripped
- 3 celery stalks, cleaved reduced down
- 2 tablespoon orange, red or green chime peppers, diced
- 1/4 cup mayonnaise
- 1/2 tablespoon rice vinegar
- 1/2 Tbsp. wasabi glue

- Salt and ichimi togarashi to taste

Directions

1. Bring a little pot of water with 1 tablespoon salt to bubble.

2. Add celery and heat up (this procedure is called whitening) for 2 minutes. Channel and wash celery in cool water. Put in a safe spot.

3. Bring another little pot of water to bubble, include shrimps and bubble for 3 minutes. Channel, wash in chilly water and put in a safe spot.

4. In a medium size blending bowl, mix mayonnaise, rice vinegar and wasabi glue together until smooth.

5. Dry the shrimps with a paper towel or hand towel, and slash them into reduced down. Add to the blending bowl.

6. Add celery and ringer peppers to the blending bowl, and mix the entirety of the fixings well. Season with salt and pepper. Serve cold.

Notes

This shrimp and celery serving of mixed greens will keep refrigerated in a hermetically sealed compartment for as long as 2 days.

Fish Steak With Tomato Relish

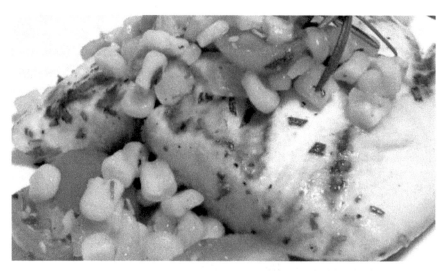

Prep Time: 5 Minutes/ Cook Time: 17 Minutes/ Total Time: 22 Minutes/

Yield: 2 1x/ Category: Main/ Cuisine: Fish, Seafood

Fixings

- 2 pounds fish steak
- 3 tablespoons additional virgin olive oil
- 1 clove garlic (finely hacked)
- 1 half quart treasure or cherry tomatoes (finely hacked)
- 1/2 medium onion (finely hacked)
- 8 leaves new basil (generally hacked)
- 1 Tbsp. sugar
- salt and pepper to taste
- lemon wedges (to serve)

Directions

1. In a dish over high warmth, include 2 tbsp olive oil, garlic and onions, and cook for 3-4 minutes, until onions are translucent. Include tomatoes and sugar, and cook for 5 minutes, or until the blend is practically similar to a sauce. Mood killer the warmth, include basil and season with salt, and pepper.

2. Use a different dish to cook the fish. Season the fish with salt and pepper on the two sides. Hold up until the dish is hot and include the staying 1 tbsp olive oil. Include fish steaks and lower the warmth to medium/high. Spread and cook until all around done (around 7 minutes). Covering the dish keeps the fish clammy, I utilize this stunt for fish, chicken and even meat; it has exactly the intended effect.

Nourishment

- Calories: 655
- Saturated Fat: 4

Stout Vegetable Soup

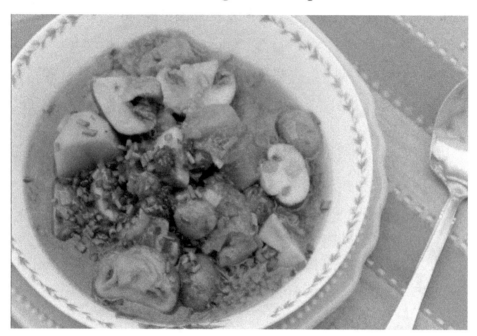

Prep Time: 15 Minutes/ Cook Time: An Hour/ Total Time: 75 Minutes/
Yield: 4 People 1x/ Category: Soup/ Cuisine: Vegetarian/ Scale 1x2x3x

Fixings

- 3 cloves garlic (finely hacked)
- 1 onion (finely hacked)
- 3 tablespoons additional virgin olive oil
- 3 medium carrots (generally cleaved)
- 2 stalks celery (generally cleaved)
- 2 turnips (generally cleaved)
- 1/4 head cabbage (generally cleaved)

- 28 oz can squashed tomatoes

- 7 cups vegetable stock

- 1/2 Tbsp. dried thyme

- dried herbs like basil oregano as well as parsley

- salt and pepper (to taste)

Directions

1. In a huge pot over high warmth, include oil, garlic, dried thyme and onions. Cook for 4-6 minutes until onions relax and turn out to be clear. Include the squashed tomatoes and mix. Include everything else; carrots, celery, turnips, cabbage, vegetable juices and dried herbs. Season with somewhat salt and bring to bubble.

2. Bring to bubble, spread and lower warmth to a stew. Cook for 25 minutes or until vegetables are cooked through. Keep an eye on your soup on occasion and mix to ensure veggies aren't consuming at the base of the pot.

3. Season with salt and pepper and serve.

Notes

This stout vegetable soup can likewise be presented with new cleaved parsley and wafers.

KETO CHAFFLE

RECIPES 2020

100+ Mouth Watering Low Carb Recipes For
Beginners. Bonus: Gluten Free Recipes For Athletes
+ Anti Aging Recipes For Women Over 50 +
Ketogenic Diet Cookbook

Serena Green

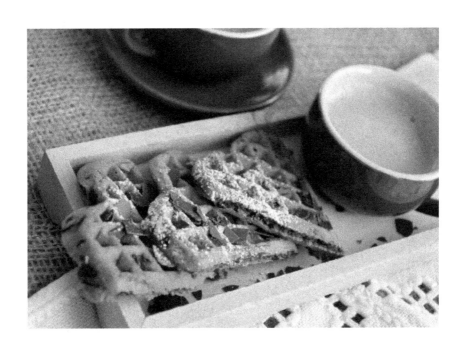

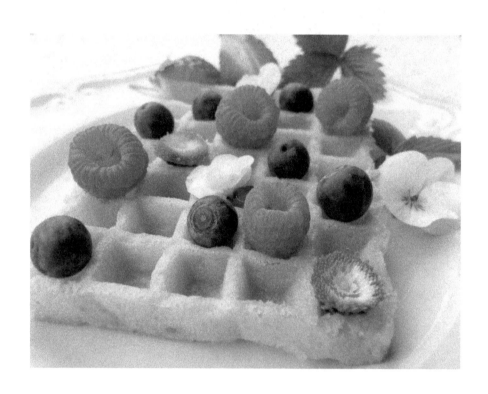

The Meaning Of Chaffle

Chaffles (short for cheddar waffles) are the most recent famous nourishment in the keto world. It's nothing unexpected — the chaffle has a great deal putting it all on the line. This straightforward keto formula is fresh, brilliant dark colored, sans sugar, low-carb, and exceptionally simple to make.

A chaffle, or cheddar waffle, is a keto waffle made with eggs and cheddar. Chaffles are turning into an extremely well known keto/low-carb nibble.

A chaffle is a waffle yet made with a cheddar base. Basically it's obliterated cheddar and an egg mix. Once in for a short time for logically fluffier recipes, it's a cream cheddar base instead of decimated cheddar. It's the a la mode new keto-pleasing bread since it's low in carbs, and it won't spike your insulin levels, causing fat accumulating.

The fundamentals are some combo of egg and cheddar; however, from here, you can riff like wild eyed. You can use an arrangement of cheeses, including cream cheddar, parmesan cheddar, etc. Some incorporate almond flour and flaxseed and getting ready powder, and others don't.

The major recipe for a chaffle contains cheddar, almond flour, and an egg. You consolidate the fixings in an astonish and pour it your waffle maker. Waffle makers are no doubt on the rising right now after this chaffle recipe exploded a couple of days back earlier. I was to some degree suspicious from the beginning intuition there was no possibility this would turn out in the wake of joining everything and pouring the hitter over the waffle. Try to sprinkle the waffle maker really well. The waffle wound up exceptional, and it was firm apparently and fragile in the inside.

You can concoct a chaffle utilizing a waffle iron or smaller than usual waffle producer. The cook time is just a couple of moments, and on the off chance that you cook the chaffle right, you end up with a fresh, gooey, flavorful bread/waffle elective.

Chaffles are turning into somewhat of a furor with supporters of the keto diet. They're less fastidious to make than most keto bread recipes and they're anything but difficult to customize. You can transform the fundamental formula for a chaffle into your own creation, running from flavorful to sweet and anything in the middle. You can likewise change the sort of cheddar you use, delivering significant changes in the flavor and surface of the chaffle. Cheddar and mozzarella cheddar are the two most regular decisions, yet you can likewise include parmesan, cream cheddar, or whatever other cheddar that melts well.

The most fundamental clarification of a Chaffle is that it's an extraordinary bread elective when on the keto diet. It copies the vibe of a waffle however Keto clients have been utilizing Chaffles in a wide range of recipes from sandwiches to sweets. There are a huge amount of Keto Chaffle Recipes out there.

The first chaffle formula starting point is obscure. Be that as it may, what a chaffle is – well, it's Keto enchantment in your mouth. It's a low carb waffle that works AWESOME for filling your requirement for bread. It just takes a couple of fixings, can be made in merely minutes and is made in a waffle creator.

It's made with cheddar, so get it? At the point when you work cheddar and waffle – you get chaffle (and you additionally get enchantment.) Well enough with the back story. Since you realize what this keto nourishment is, how about we make one and let you see with your own eyes how astounding this keto waffle is.

What Is Needed To Prepare A Chaffle

- 1 tremendous egg
- 1/2 c. Cheddar
- 2 tablespoons of almond flour

How To Prepare A Chaffle

There are a few hints, techniques and approaches you'll need to know to make your chaffles particularly fresh.

Most importantly, don't eat your chaffles directly out of the waffle iron. They'll be wet and eggy from the outset, however on the off chance that you let them sit for 3-4 minutes, they'll fresh right up.

Second, for extra fresh chaffles, you can include an additional layer of destroyed cheddar (or another cheddar that gets firm, similar to parmesan) to the two sides of the waffle producer's surface. Set out the destroyed cheddar, pour in the hitter, put more cheddar on top, and afterward cook the chaffle typically. You'll wind up with firm, sautéed bits of cheddar installed in the outside of the chaffle.

Everyone is going looney tunes, asking, "How might I make these?!" This is the game plan The principal recipe on what and how. The fundamental equation consolidates crushed cheddar and an egg; however, there are tremendous measures of add-ins you can use to change the flavor! You will make a direct chaffle hitter and cook it in a waffle maker!

To make a chaffle equation, you will fundamentally join two or three fixings and cook it in a waffle maker to make a perfect work of art everyone will value!

5. Preheat your waffle maker if it requires preheating.
6. Whisk together the egg, cheddar, almond flour, and setting up the soda pop in a bowl until all-around joined.
7. Shower the waffle maker with a cooking sprinkle and pour the chaffle player over the waffle maker. Close and let the waffle for 3 to 4 minutes. My waffle maker has it's own customized clock setting.
8. Remove the waffle from the waffle press and welcome it.

The Waffle Tools To Make Easy Keto Chaffles

A standard waffle creator will deliver a chaffle that appears as though the universally adored round solidified toaster waffles, which is flawless as keto bread for sandwiches, a bun for burgers, or even a shell for tacos. One famous brand is the Dash smaller than expected waffle creator, which is entirely reasonable and makes slender, fresh chaffles.

A Belgian waffle creator makes thicker waffles with profound scores. That is incredible for typical waffle-production, however it isn't perfect for chaffles. They end up less fresh, with a greater amount of an omelet-like consistency. Your most logical option is to get a standard waffle producer.

How To Eat Chaffles

There are a great deal of famous approaches to eat chaffles.

- Plain. Chaffles are incredible all alone as a morning meal nourishment. You can serve them up close by bacon, eggs, avocado, and other standard keto breakfast passage.
- Keto chaffle sandwich. Make two chaffles and use them as bread for your preferred sandwich. Chaffles are extraordinary as the bread for BLTs, turkey clubs, breakfast sandwiches, or some other keto-accommodating sandwich.
- Chaffle dessert. Attempt one of the sweet chaffle varieties recorded underneath and present with keto maple syrup or your most loved keto frozen yogurt.

The Different Type Of Waffle Maker Needed To Make A Chaffle

By far most genuinely like to use a Dash Mini Waffle Maker; however, you can use any waffle maker you have. There is a wide scope of waffle makers.

Honestly, you in all likelihood have one in the back of your kitchen organizers that you haven't used in quite a while. Most by far who don't have a waffle maker may even find one at a Goodwill or Salvation Army. There's no absence of these helpful kitchen gadgets in these reused stores.

The Various Types Of Basic Keto Chaffle Recipes

Keto Chaffle Recipes eBook Cookbook for beginners 2020, includes delicious and appealing keto recipes for each flavor palette.

5. Basic Chaffle Recipes
6. Savory Chaffle Recipes
7. Sweet Chaffle Recipes
8. Chaffle Cake Recipes

Various Cheeses

Cheddar, mozzarella, parmesan, cream cheddar, colby jack — any cheddar that melts well will work with a chaffle. Distinctive cheddar produce various flavors and somewhat various surfaces. Attempt a couple and locate your top choice.

Sweet Chaffles

Utilize a nonpartisan cheddar like mozzarella or cream cheddar, at that point include a touch of your most loved keto sugar to the hitter before you cook it. You can likewise chocolate chips or low-sugar fruits like blueberries or strawberries. Top with keto frozen yogurt or keto whipped cream for a delectable chaffle dessert.

Exquisite Chaffles

Include exquisite fixings like herbs and flavors to your chaffle. For a pizza chaffle, include oregano, garlic powder, and diced pepperoni in the hitter, with tomato sauce and additional cheddar on top. Or on the other hand you could utilize cream cheddar and add everything bagel flavoring to the player for an everything bagel chaffle. Present with more cream cheddar on top, tricks, onions, and smoked salmon.

Rules On How To Make The Best Chaffles

17. Tolerance. That is the best tip. They don't take long, yet if you need a new keto waffle, you are just should be to some degree patient and let it take the 5-7 minutes that it takes to new up. Precisely when you trust it's done? Permit it one greater minute or two. Make an effort not to flood.

18. Layering. In the event that you're making a chaffle with cheddar, the best way to deal with do this is to layer cheddar at the base, pour in a tablespoon or so of egg, and a short time later top with cheddar again. It's the firm cheddar on the base and top that will make them new.

19. Shallow waffles. If you need new waffles, the shallower the waffle iron, the more straightforward/faster it is to new up the chaffle.

20. No over-burdening. Stuffed chaffle makers… well, they flood clearly. Which makes colossal destruction! So when in doubt,

under fill rather than pressing. Near 1/4 cup of TOTAL fixings in a steady progression.

21. Crush it. I've thought about others using press bottles so they can get just a little egg into the small scale waffle maker.

22. Simple cleanup. I like to use a wet paper towel when the waffle iron is warm, to make cleanup straightforward. Not hot, however, obviously! Essentially warm.

23. Brush it. I've found toothbrush works outstandingly to clean between the waffle iron teeth. You can in like manner endeavor this wipe cleaner, which I also use to clean the little region on the edge of my Instant Pot.

24. No looking. I can tell you from LOTS of individual experience, that opening the waffle iron at normal interims "just to check" doesn't hep the chaffle cook any speedier. Your most consistent choice is to not using any and all means open it for 4-5 minutes.

25. No steaming. on the off chance that you're using the Dash small, the little blue light goes out when it's commonly cooked, yet most importantly, the chaffle stops steaming to such a degree. That is a better than average sign that it's done.

26. Get hot. Hold up until the waffle iron is hot before you incorporate fixings, and they're essentially less slanted to adhere and a lot easier to clean up.

27. Tangle it. Alright, so about that flood. I do find that it unfolds more routinely than I may need! One thing that has made

cleanup more straightforward for me has been to put a silicone trivet underneath.

28. Cut or shred. I understand most recipes out there suggest demolished cheddar, yet I have better karma with the slimmest cut of cheddar I can buy. I find it crisps essentially speedier.

29. Not really eggy. If you find your chaffles too eggy, use egg white as opposed to the whole egg.

30. Not really gooey. In case you need them to taste less gooey, endeavor mozzarella cheddar.

31. Fresh Cooling. License the chaffles to cool before eating. They get crisper as they cool, so take the necessary steps not to stuff the hot chaffle into your mouth right away.

32. Make parts. Make enough to share, and everyone will require them, whether or not they're keto or not.

Chaffles Nutrition and Carb Count

You'll get two chaffles out of an enormous egg and about a large portion of a cup of cheddar. Contingent upon the cheddar you use, your calories and net carb check will change a tad. Yet, as a rule, expecting you utilize genuine, entire milk cheddar like cheddar or mozzarella (rather than cream cheddar or American cheddar), chaffles are totally sans carb. A normal serving size of two chaffles contains generally:

- 300 calories
- 0g all out carbs
- 0g net carbs

- 20g protein

- 23g fat

As should be obvious, chaffles are about as keto as a formula can be: high-fat, high-protein, and zero-carb. They even work on the flesh eater diet, if you eat cheddar.

The Best Keto Chaffle Recipes To Try

Including recipes for some work of art, high-carb top picks that have been adjusted to be "fat bombs," which help keep your macros in balance, just as keep you from desiring every one of the things you, for the most part, can't eat when you're attempting to get more fit.

A considerable amount of the in excess of 200 recipes require close to 10 to 15 minutes of planning time, and they taste as scrumptious and liberal as they sound–what about Chocolate Peanut Butter Pops, Mocha Cheesecake, or Almond Butter Bombs?

Keto Chaffle Recipe

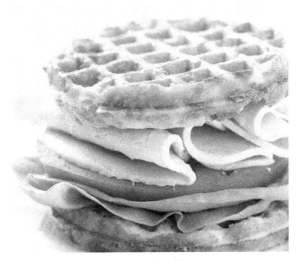

Keto chaffles are the most recent new rage! The entire formula is just 3 net carbs all out.

Ingredients

- 1 huge egg
- 1/2 c. Cheddar
- 2 tablespoons of almond flour

Rich And Creamy Chaffles Recipe

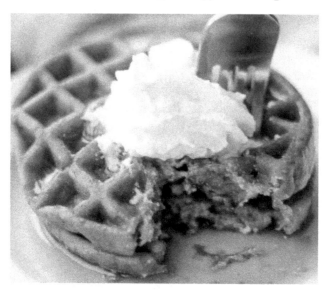

- 2 eggs
- 1 cup destroyed mozzarella
- 2 tablespoons almond flour
- 2 tablespoons cream cheddar
- 3/4 Tbsp. preparing power
- 3 tablespoons water (discretionary)
- Makes 6 waffles.

Zucchini Chuffles | Zuffles Recipe

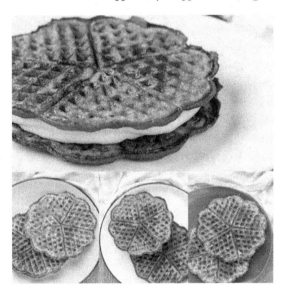

- 1 little zucchini, ground
- 1 egg
- 1 tablespoon parmesan
- Small bunch of destroyed mozzarella
- Basil and pepper to taste
- Mix all together and cook in a full-size waffle producer.
- Makes 2 full-size waffles and a meager zaffle.

Light And Crispy Chaffles Recipe

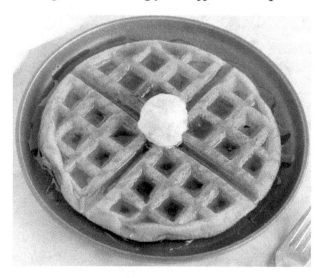

- 1 egg

- 1/3 cup cheddar

- 1/4 Tbsp. heating powder

- 1/2 Tbsp. ground flaxseed

- Shredded parmesan cheddar on top and base.

- Stir and cook in a mini waffle iron until fresh.

Keto Sausage Ball

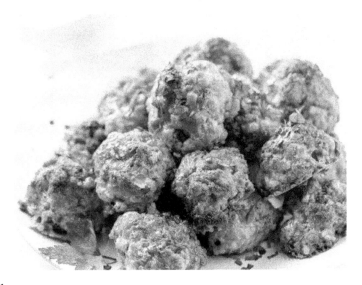

Portrayal

Keto Sausage Balls just contain four straightforward ingredients and make an extraordinary canapé or bite. They just contain 1 net carb and can without much of a stretch fit into your low carb or keto way of life.

Ingredients

- 2 cups of almond flour
- 2 cups of cheddar
- 1 pound of pork wiener
- 8 oz of cream cheddar

Fat Head Pizza Crust

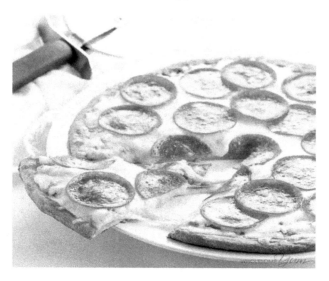

Ingredients

- 1 1/2 cups destroyed mozzarella
- 3/4 cup almond flour
- 2 tablespoons of cream cheddar, cubed
- 1 egg
- garlic powder, onion powder, and blended herbs for flavoring *see notes

Chicken Stuffed Avocado

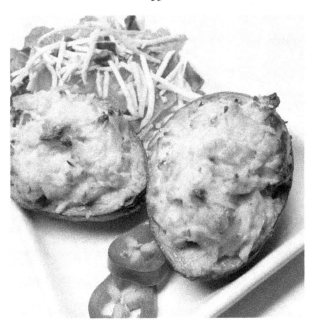

Portrayal

Wild ox Chicken Stuffed Avocado is a brisk formula utilizing stovetop bison chicken plunge and avocados. Making wild ox chicken plunge is extremely simple utilizing a stovetop too.

Ingredients

- 2 5 oz jars of chicken, depleted
- 2 tablespoons of whipped cream cheddar
- 2 tsp of dry Ranch flavoring blend
- ¼ cup of sans fat cheddar (utilize full fat with keto or low carb)
- 2 tablespoons of Frank's Buffalo Wing Sauce
- 1 medium avocado

Almond Flour Blueberry Pancakes

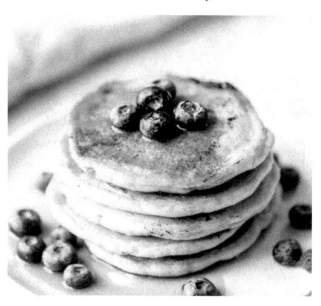

Depiction

Basic almond flour flapjacks made with just 6 ingredients. 2 net carbs per hotcake!

Ingredients

- 2 huge eggs
- ⅓ cup unsweetened almond milk
- 1 Tbsp. vanilla concentrate
- 1 ¼ cup fine almond flour (utilized Bob's, Red Mill)
- ¼ Tbsp. preparing pop
- Touch of salt
- Spread for lubing the skillet

Boston Brown Bread Recipe

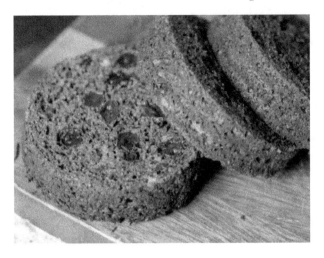

Ingredients

- 1 Egg
- 1 cup buttermilk, or 1 cup milk with 1 tablespoon vinegar blended in
- 1/4 cup Molasses
- 1/4 cup Sugar
- 1 tablespoon Oil
- 1.5 cups Whole Wheat Flour
- 1/2 cup Cornmeal
- 2 Tbsp.s Baking Powder
- 1 Tbsp. Ground Allspice
- 1/2 cup slashed pecans
- 1/4 cup Raisins

Keto Cheese Muffins

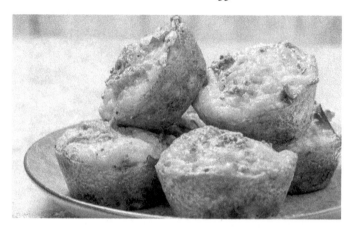

Ingredients

- Vegetable oil for lubing the skillet
- 1 cup (112 g) Superfine Almond Flour
- 1/2 cup (85 g) Black Chia Seeds
- 2 Tbsp.s (2 Tbsp.s) Baking Powder
- 1/2 Tbsp. (118.29 g) granulated garlic
- 4 enormous (4 huge) Eggs
- 1/4 cup (56.75 g) softened margarine
- 1/2 cup (56.5 g) ground cheddar

Air Fryer Breaded Chicken Wings

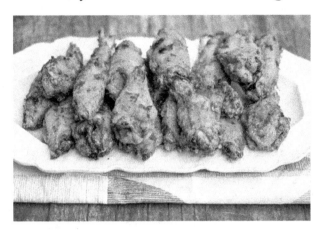

Ingredients

- 1 pound (453.59 g) chicken wings

- 3 tablespoons (3 tablespoons) Vegetable Oil

- 1/2 cup (62.5 g) All-Purpose Flour

- 1/2 Tbsp. (0.5 Tbsp.) Smoked Paprika

- 1/2 Tbsp. (0.5 Tbsp.s) Garlic Powder

- 1/2 Tbsp. (0.5 Tbsp.) Salt

- 1/2 Tbsp. (0.5 Tbsp.s) naturally squashed peppercorn

One Step Brazilian Pao De Queijo Brazilian Cheese Bread

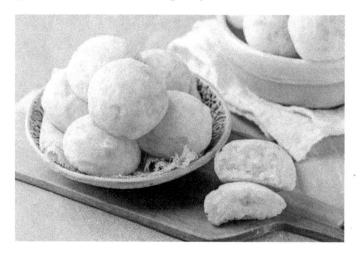

Ingredients

- 1 cup (244 g) Whole Milk
- 1/2 cup (112 g) Oil
- 1 Tbsp. (1 Tbsp.) Salt
- 2 cups (240 g) Tapioca Flour
- 2 (2) Eggs
- 1.5 cups (150 g) destroyed parmesan cheddar

Keto Zucchini Walnut Bread

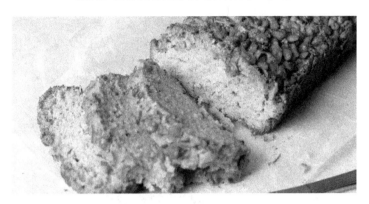

Need to make a Keto Zucchini Bread, you'll be super eager to eat and serve to other people? This formula with pecans is great!

Ingredients

- 1/2 cup (0.5 g) Truvia
- 3 (3) Eggs
- 1/2 cup (109 g) Ghee or Oil
- 1.5 cups (168 g) Superfine Almond Flour
- 1/2 cups (60 g) coconut flour
- 1 Tbsp. (1 Tbsp.) Baking Powder
- 1 Tbsp. (1 Tbsp.) Baking Soda
- 1/2 Tbsp. (0.5 Tbsp.s) Ground Cinnamon
- 1/4 Tbsp. Ground Nutmeg
- 1/2 cup (250 g) Unsweetened Almond Milk
- 2 cups (248 g) destroyed zucchini
- 1 cup (117 g) cleaved pecans

Keto Bread | Nut And Seed Bread

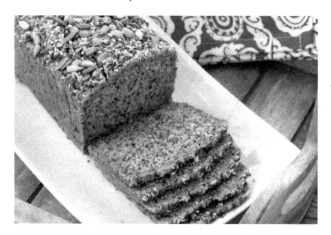

Ingredients

3 cups blended nuts and seeds left entire for instance

- 1/2 cup (61.5 g) pistachios
- 1/2 cup (71.5 g) almonds
- 1/2 cup (84 g) flaxseed
- 1/2 cup (58.5 g) pecans
- 1/2 cup (75 g) Sesame Seeds
- 1/2 cup (64.5 g) cashews

Different Ingredients

- 3 (3) Eggs
- 1/4 cup (56 ml) Oil
- 1/3 tsp (0.33 tsp) Salt

One Step Brazilian Pao De Queijo Brazilian Cheese Bread

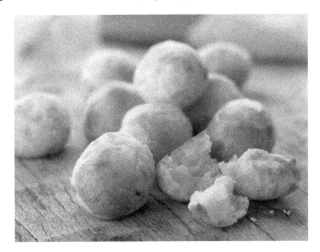

Ingredients

- 1 cup (244 g) Whole Milk
- 1/2 cup (112 g) Oil
- 1 Tbsp. (1 Tbsp.) Salt
- 2 cups (240 g) Tapioca Flour
- 2 (2) Eggs
- 1.5 cups (150 g) destroyed parmesan cheddar

Sweet Cream Truffles

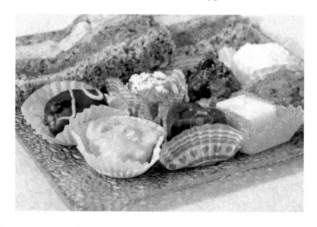

Ingredients

For the Truffle Center

- 2 cups (476 g) Heavy Whipping Cream
- 1/2 cup (91 g) powdered Swerve
- For the Chocolate Coating
- 2 ounces (56.7 g) Sugar-Free Chocolate Chips
- 1 tablespoon (1 tablespoon) Butter

Keto Milky Bears| Gummy Bear Recipe

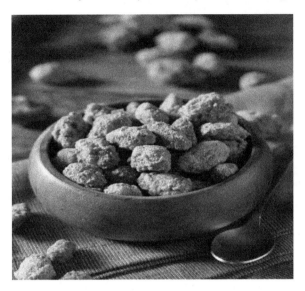

These Keto Milky Bears are a fabulous sweet treat that won't take you out of ketosis. They're low carb, without gluten thus great you can't simply eat one! Obviously superior to normal keto sticky bears.

Ingredients

- 1 13.5 ounces (1) Full-Fat Coconut Milk
- 2 bundles (2) unflavored gelatin, (3 tablespoons)
- 1/4 cup (62.5 g) Water
- 3 tablespoons (3 tablespoons) Truvia
- 2-3 drops (2) Pandan Extract

Keto Coconut Panna Cotta

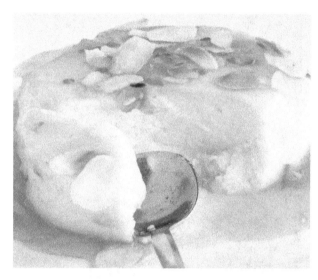

This straightforward Coconut Panna Cotta formula so sweet, smooth, and yummy that it will get one of your go-to pastries! Also, it's low carb and dairy-free!

Ingredients

- 1/2 cup cold water
- 1 bundle unflavored gelatin, 1/4 oz or 2.5 Tbsp.s
- 13.5 ounces Full-Fat Coconut Milk
- 1/8 cup Truvia
- 1 Tbsp. unadulterated vanilla concentrate or coconut extricate

Keto Chocolate Cheesecake Brownies

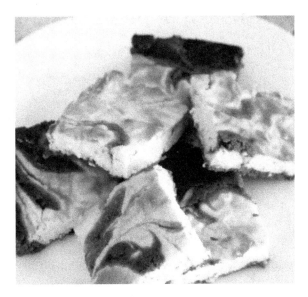

These Keto Chocolate Cheesecake Brownies are a chocolate cheesecake darlings dream! They're so acceptable you won't have the option to tell their low carb!

Ingredients

For the Brownie Batter

- 1/2 cup (90 g) Sugar-Free Chocolate Chips
- 1/2 cup (113.5 g) Butter
- 3 (3) Eggs
- 1/4 cup (0.25 g) Truvia, or other sugar
- 1 Tbsp. (1 Tbsp.) vanilla concentrate
- For the Cheesecake Batter
- 8 ounces (226.8 g) Cream Cheese, cubed and relaxed

- 1 (1) Egg
- 3 tablespoons (3 tablespoons) Truvia, or other sugar
- 1 Tbsp. (1 Tbsp.) vanilla concentrate

Keto Pie Crust

This 3-ingredient pat out Keto Pie Crust formula is a keto dieter's dream! No compelling reason to make crustless pies so as to keep it low carb. It's totally keto and vegan.

Ingredients

- 1 cup (112 g) Superfine Almond Flour
- 2 tablespoons (2 tablespoons) powdered Swerve
- 1/4 cup (54.5 g) Melted Coconut Oil

Keto Maple Pecan Blondies

These Keto Maple Pecan Blondies are the ideal sweet treat to fulfill your sweet tooth. They're wonderfully rich and shockingly low carb!

Ingredients

- 1 cup (112 g) Superfine Almond Flour
- 1/4 cup (30 g) coconut flour
- 2 Tbsp.s (2 Tbsp.s) Baking Powder
- 1/2 cup (91 g) Swerve
- 1/2 cup (113.5 g) Butter, softened
- 3 (3) Eggs
- 1 Tbsp. (1 Tbsp.) maple separate

- 3/4 cup (87.75 g) slashed pecans

Keto Lasagna

Make this simple Keto Lasagna formula in your air fryer utilizing zucchini rather than conventional pasta noodles. It's so acceptable you won't miss the pasta!

Ingredients

- 1 cup marinara sauce
- 1 zucchini, cut into long, flimsy cuts
- For Meat Layer
- 1 cup finely slashed yellow onion
- 1 Tbsp. Minced Garlic
- 1/2 pound-mass hot or mellow Italian frankfurter
- 1/2 cup ricotta cheddar
- 1/2 cup destroyed mozzarella cheddar
- 1/2 cup destroyed parmesan,, isolated
- 1 Egg
- 1/2 Tbsp. Garlic, minced
- 1/2 Tbsp. Italian Seasoning
- 1/2 Tbsp. Ground Black Pepper

Keto Almond Phirni Kheer

This Keto Almond Phirni Kheer is a heavenly Indian pastry formula that you're going to experience passionate feelings for! In addition, it is tasty, it's low carb as well!

Ingredients

- 3/4 cup (178.5 g) Heavy Whipping Cream
- 1 cup (250 g) Unsweetened Almond Milk
- 1/2 cup (56 g) Superfine Almond Flour
- 2 tablespoons (2 tablespoons) Truvia
- 1/2-1 Tbsp. (0.5 Tbsp.s) Ground Cardamom
- 2-3 (2) Saffron Strands, squashed

Tomato Eggplant Soup

This is such an incredible vegan Tomato Eggplant Soup formula! Empty everything into your Instant Pot, and you'll have a bowl of great Mediterranean soup for supper in less than 30 minutes.

Ingredients

- 3 tablespoons Oil
- 2 tablespoons Minced Garlic
- 4 cups Eggplant, hacked
- 2 cups Tomatoes, hacked, or 1 14.5 ounce canned tomatoes, depleted
- 1 cup Onion, hacked

- 1 cup chime pepper, cleaved
- 1/2 cup Water
- 1 Tbsp. salt
- 1 Tbsp. Ground Black Pepper
- For Finishing
- 1/4 cup Basil, hacked

Hamburger Kheema Meatloaf

Tired of normal meatloaf? Can't manage one more night of tacos to go through that ground hamburger? Make proper acquaintance with air fryer keto Indian Kheema meatloaf! Appreciate Indian food in a manner you may be comfortable with by making this Beef Kheema Meatloaf in your Air Fryer.

Ingredients

- 1 lb Lean Ground Beef
- 2 Eggs
- 1 cup Onion, diced
- 1/4 cup Cilantro, hacked
- 1 tbsp minced ginger
- 1 tbsp Minced Garlic
- 2 tsp Garam Masala
- 1 tsp Salt
- 1 tsp Turmeric
- 1 tsp cayenne

- 1/2 tsp Ground Cinnamon
- 1/8 tsp Ground Cardamom

Weight Cooker Low Carb Wontons

Make these low carb wontons in your Instant pot, for the most delicate and succulent low carb wontons you've at any point had. Make these wontons without any wrappers, yet the entirety of the flavor of customary wontons.

Ingredients

- 1 pound (453.59 g) ground pork
- 1/4 cup (25 g) Green Onions, green and white parts blended
- 1/4 cup (4 g) Chopped Cilantro or Parsley
- 2 Tbsp.s (2 Tbsp.s) Soy Sauce
- 1 Tbsp. (1 Tbsp.) Oyster sauce
- 1 Tbsp. (1 Tbsp.) Ground Black Pepper
- ½ Tbsp. (0.5 Tbsp.) Salt
- 1 tablespoon (1 tablespoon) minced ginger
- 1 tablespoon (1 tablespoon) Minced Garlic
- 2 (2) Eggs

Keto Chicken Biryani

This Low Carb Chicken Biryani formula is Low-Carb Indian Food at it's ideal. Cauliflower and ground chicken make up this fiery, heavenly low carb formula.

Ingredients

For Chicken

- 1 Tbsp. Ghee
- 1 pound Ground Chicken
- 1 Tbsp. salt
- 1/2 Tbsp. Turmeric
- 1 Tbsp. Garam Masala
- 1/2 Tbsp. Ground Coriander
- 1/4 Tbsp. Ground Cumin

Vegetables

- 1 Tbsp. Ghee
- 1 Red Onion, cut meager
- 1 Jalapeño pepper, diced
- 1 Tbsp. ginger-garlic glue, (or 1/2 Tbsp.s minced garlic, 1/2 Tbsp.s minced ginger)
- 1/2 cup Water
- 1/2 cup Cilantro, slashed
- 1/4 cup mint leaves, slashed
- 2 cups cauliflower, riced

Moment Pot Cauliflower "Macintosh" And Cheese Low Carb

Moment Pot Low Carb Keto Cauliflower and Cheese is a velvety, delightful side dish that you can make in your weight cooker for a definitive low carb comfort food!

Ingredients

- 2 cups (214 g) cauliflower, riced
- 2 tablespoon (2 tablespoons) Cream Cheese
- 1/2 cup (56.5 g) destroyed sharp cheddar
- 1/2 Tbsp. (0.5 Tbsp.) Salt
- 1/2 Tbsp. (0.5 Tbsp.s) Ground Black Pepper

Keto Ham And Bean Soup

No compelling reason to miss beans on a low carb diet. This Keto Ham and Bean Soup formula utilize a mystery, keto bean substitute that preferences simply like the genuine article.

Ingredients

- 1 cup (186 g) dried dark soybeans, doused to yield 2 cups beans
- 1 cup (160 g) onions, slashed
- 1 cup (101 g) slashed celery
- 4 cloves (4 cloves) Minced Garlic
- 1 Tbsp. (1 Tbsp.) Dried Oregano
- .5 to 1 Tbsp. salt
- 1 Tbsp. (1 Tbsp.) Cajun Seasoning
- 1 Tbsp. (1 Tbsp.) Liquid Smoke
- 2 Tbsp.s (2 Tbsp.s) Tony Chachere's universally handy flavoring
- 1 Tbsp. (1 Tbsp.) Louisiana Hot sauce
- 1 (1) substantial ham bone or 2 smoked ham sells
- 2 cups (280 g) slashed ham

- 2 cups (16.91 floz) Water

Simple Mango Cardamom Pannacotta

Low Carb Panna Cotta sets up rapidly and is a reviving summer dessert. Delicious, rich panna cotta joined with sweet mango.

Ingredients

- 1 tablespoon (1 tablespoon) unflavored gelatin
- 2 cups (488 g) Fairlife entire milk, (separated)
- 1 cup (165 g) mango
- 1 cup (238 g) Heavy Whipping Cream
- 1/2 cup (91 g) Swerve, or other sugar
- 1 Tbsp. (1 Tbsp.) Ground Cardamom

Smooth Shrimp Scampi

Simple Low Carb Keto Creamy Shrimp Scampi from your moment pot or weight cooker, this one cooks quick! Put it over some low carb noodles for a snappy supper.

Ingredients

- 2 tablespoons Butter
- 1 pound Shrimp, solidified
- 4 cloves Garlic, minced
- 1/4-1/2 Tbsp.s Red Pepper Flakes
- 1/2 Tbsp.s Smoked Paprika
- 2 cups Carbanada low carb pasta, (uncooked)

- 1 cup Chicken Broth

- 1/2 cup Half and Half

- 1/2 cup Parmesan Cheese

- Salt, to taste

- Ground Black Pepper, to taste

Moment Pot Spaghetti Squash

When you make Spaghetti squash in the Instant pot, you will never make it another way. Eight minutes under tension, without cutting the squash, and you have the ideal low carb or veggie lover side dish.

Ingredients

- 1 Large Spaghetti Squash

- 1.5 cups Water, for the Instant Pot

Tomato Eggplant Soup

This is such an extraordinary vegan Tomato Eggplant Soup formula! Empty everything into your Instant Pot, and you'll have a magnificent Mediterranean soup for supper in less than 30 minutes.

Ingredients

- 3 tablespoons Oil

- 2 tablespoons Minced Garlic

- 4 cups Eggplant, slashed

- 2 cups Tomatoes, slashed, or 1 14.5 ounce canned tomatoes, depleted

- 1 cup Onion, slashed

- 1 cup ringer pepper, cleaved

- 1/2 cup Water

- 1 Tbsp. salt

- 1 Tbsp. Ground Black Pepper

Moment Pot Sauerkraut Soup Recipe

Utilize your Instant Pot to make this flavorful, low-carb Sauerkraut Soup formula! It's a simple dump and cooks formula that cooks in a short time.

Ingredients

- 1 cup dried cannellini beans, drenched medium-term and depleted

- 14 oz smoked frankfurters, cut down the middle longwise, and afterward cut into 1-inch pieces

- 1 cup sauerkraut with brackish water

- 3 Bay Leaves

- 1 cup onions, slashed

- 1 tablespoon Minced Garlic

- 1 Tbsp. Salt

- 1 Tbsp. Ground Black Pepper

- 4 cups Water

Chicken And Mushrooms Recipe

If you need to make a Chicken and Mushrooms Recipe, however, would prefer not to utilize canned soup, have I got only the thing for you! It's Keto and Instant Pot also!

Ingredients

- 2 tablespoons (2 tablespoons) Butter
- 1 cup (160 g) Sliced Onions
- 6 (6) Garlic Cloves, cut slender
- 1 cup (186 g) Mushrooms, cut into quarters
- 1 lb (453.59 g) Boneless Skinless Chicken Thighs
- 4 cups (120 g) infant spinach
- 2 tablespoons (2 tablespoons) Water
- 1 Tbsp.ful of Dried Thyme, or 3-4 sprigs crisp thyme
- 1 Tbsp. (1 Tbsp.) Salt
- 1 Tbsp.ful of Ground Black Pepper
- For Finishing
- 1/2 cup (119 g) Heavy Whipping Cream
- 1 tablespoon (1 tablespoon) lemon juice

Keto Shrimp Scampi

8 minutes from beginning to end to make this air fryer keto low carb shrimp scampi. So easy to make, so heavenly, you will have a hard time believing it.

Ingredients

- 4 tablespoons (4 tablespoons) Butter
- 1 tablespoon (1 tablespoon) lemon juice
- 1 tablespoon (1 tablespoon) Minced Garlic
- 2 Tbsp.s (2 Tbsp.s) Red Pepper Flakes
- 1 tablespoon (1 tablespoon) hacked chives, or 1 Tbsp. dried chives
- 1 tablespoon (1 tablespoon) hacked crisp basil, or 1 Tbsp. dried basil
- 2 tablespoons of Chicken Stock, (or white wine)
- 1 lb (453.59 g) defrosted shrimp, (21-25 check)

Essential Indian Curry Recipe | Pressure Cooker Curry Recipe

This Basic Indian Curry is a tasty customary Indian curry formula made in the Instant Pot! This curry formula is low-carb and stuffed with Indian flavor.

Ingredients

- 1 pound (453.59 g) Boneless Pork Shoulder, diced into 2 inch 3D squares
- 1.5 cups (240 g) onions, hacked
- 1 cup (242 g) Canned Tomatoes, undrained
- 1 tablespoon (1 tablespoon) Minced Garlic
- 1 tablespoon minced ginger
- 2 Tbsp.s (2 Tbsp.s) Garam Masala, separated
- 1 Tbsp. (1 Tbsp.) Salt

- 1 Tbsp. (1 Tbsp.) Turmeric

- 1/4-1 Tbsp. (0.25 Tbsp.) Cayenne

- 2 tablespoons (2 tablespoons) Water

Chicken Tikka Masala

Make simple, real Chicken Tikka Masala comfortable in your Instant Pot or weight cooker! It's by a wide margin the simplest method to make Chicken Tikka Masala.

Ingredients

Marinate the chicken

- 1 ½ pound (680.39 g) Boneless Skinless Chicken Thighs, (bosom or thighs), cut into enormous pieces

- ½ cups (100 g) Greek Yogurt

- 4 cloves (4 cloves) Garlic, minced

- 2 Tbsp.s (2 Tbsp.s) minced ginger, minced

- ½ Tbsp. (0.5 Tbsp.) Turmeric

- ¼ Tbsp. (0.25 Tbsp.) Cayenne

- ½ Tbsp. (0.5 Tbsp.s) Smoked Paprika, for shading and a somewhat smoky taste

- 1 Tbsp. (1 Tbsp.) Salt

- 1 Tbsp. (1 Tbsp.) Garam Masala

- 1/2 Tbsp. (0.5 Tbsp.s) Ground Cumin

- 1 Tbsp. (1 Tbsp.) Liquid Smoke, (overlook if inaccessible)

Simple Traditional Keto Chaffle

Ingredients

- 1 Egg
- 1/2 cup Shredded Cheddar Cheese

Directions

- Preheat mini waffle creator.
- In a cucp, whisk the egg until beaten.
- Add destroyed cheddar and mix to consolidate.
- When the waffle creator is warmed, cautiously pour 1/2 of the hitter in the waffle producer and close the top. Permit to cook for 3-5 minutes.
- Carefully expel from the waffle producer and put in a safe spot for 2-3 minutes to fresh up.
- Repeat guidelines again for the second chaffle.

Keto Strawberry Shortcake Chaffle

Ingredients

- 1 Egg
- 1 tbsp Heavy Whipping Cream
- 1 tsp Coconut Flour
- 2 tbsp Lakanto Golden Sweetener (Use butter together for 20% off)
- 1/2 tsp Cake Batter Extract
- 1/4 tsp Baking powder

Keto Pumpkin Cheesecake Chaffle

Ingredients

Pumpkin Chaffle

- 1 Egg

- 1/2 cup Mozzarella Cheese

- 1 1/2 tbsp Pumpkin Puree (100% pumpkin)

- 1 tbsp Almond Flour

- 1 tbsp Lakanto Golden Sweetener, or decision of sugar

- 2 tsp Heavy Cream

- 1 tsp Cream Cheese, relaxed

- 1/2 tsp Pumpkin Spice

- 1/2 tsp Baking Powder

- 1/2 tsp Vanilla

- 1 tsp Choczero Maple Syrup or 1/8 tsp Maple Extract

Tasty Keto Pizza Chaffle Recipe

Ingredients

Chaffle Crust

- 1 Egg

- 1/2 cup Mozzarella Cheese

- 1 tsp Coconut Flour

- 1/4 tsp Baking Powder

- 1/8 tsp Garlic Powder

- 1/8 tsp Italian Seasoning
- Pinch of Salt

Pizza Topping

- 1 tbsp Rao's Marinara Sauce
- 1/2 cup Mozzarella Cheese
- 3 Pepperoni's, cut into four
- Shredded Parmesan Cheese, discretionary
- Parsley, discretionary

Best Oreo Keto Chaffles

Ingredients

Chocolate Chaffle

- 1 Egg
- 1 1/2 tbsp Unsweetened Cocoa
- 2 tbsp Lakanto Monkfruit, or decision of sugar
- 1 tbsp Heavy Cream
- 1 tsp Coconut Flour
- 1/2 tsp Baking Powder
- 1/2 tsp Vanilla

Filling

- Whipped Cream (interchange icing formula in notes beneath)

Guidelines

- Preheat mini waffle producer.

- In a small bowl, join all chaffle ingredients.
- Pour a portion of the chaffle blend into the focal point of the waffle iron. Permit to cook for 3-5 minutes.

Keto Peanut Butter Cup Chaffle

Ingredients

Chaffle

- 1 Egg
- 1 tbsp Heavy Cream
- 1 tbsp Unsweetened Cocoa
- 1 tbsp Lakanto Powdered Sweetener
- 1 tsp Coconut Flour
- 1/2 tsp Vanilla Extract
- 1/2 Cake Batter Flavor (we utilize this)
- 1/4 tsp Baking Powder

Nutty spread FILLING

- 3 tbsp All regular Peanut Butter
- 2 tsp Lakanto Powdered Sweetener
- 2 tbsp Heavy Cream

Keto Snickerdoodle Chaffle

Ingredients

- 1 Egg
- 1/2 cup Mozzarella Cheese

- 2 tbsp Almond Flour
- 1 tbsp Lakanto Golden Sweetener
- 1/2 tsp Vanilla Extract
- 1/4 tsp Cinnamon
- 1/2 tsp Baking Powder
- 1/4 tsp Cream of tartar, discretionary

Covering

- 1 tbsp Butter
- 2 tbsp Lakanto Classic Sweetener
- 1/2 tsp Cinnamon

Guidelines

- Preheat your mini waffle producer.
- In a little bowl, join all chaffle ingredients.
- Pour a portion of the chaffle blend on to the focal point of the waffle iron. Permit to cook for 3-5 minutes.
- Carefully expel and rehash for the second chaffle. Permit chaffles to cool so they fresh.
- In a little bowl, consolidate sugar and cinnamon for covering.
- Melt spread in a little microwave-safe bowl and brush the chaffles with the margarine.
- Sprinkle sugar and cinnamon blend on the two sides of the chaffles once they're brushed with margarine.

White Bread Keto Chaffle | Wonder Bread Chaffle

Ingredients

- 1 Egg
- 3 tbsp Almond Flour
- 1 tbsp Mayonnaise
- 1/4 tsp Baking Powder
- 1 tsp Water

Guidelines

- Preheat mini waffle producer.
- In a cup, whisk the egg until beaten.
- Add almond flour, mayonnaise, heating powder, and water.
- When the waffle producer is warmed, cautiously pour 1/2 of the hitter in the waffle creator and close the top. Permit to cook for 3-5 minutes.
- Carefully expel from the waffle creator and put in a safe spot for 2-3 minutes to fresh up.
- Repeat directions again for the second chaffle.

Best Oreo Keto Chaffles

Ingredients

Chocolate Chaffle

- 1 Egg
- 1 1/2 tbsp Unsweetened Cocoa

- 2 tbsp Lakanto Monkfruit, or decision of sugar
- 1 tbsp Heavy Cream
- 1 tsp Coconut Flour
- 1/2 tsp Baking Powder
- 1/2 tsp Vanilla

FILLING

- Whipped Cream (exchange icing formula in notes beneath)

Guidelines

- Preheat mini waffle producer.
- In a small bowl, join all chaffle ingredients.
- Pour a portion of the chaffle blend into the focal point of the waffle iron. Permit to cook for 3-5 minutes.

Keto Chocolate Chip Chaffle Keto Recipe

Ingredients

- 1 egg
- 1 tbsp substantial whipping cream
- 1/2 tsp coconut flour
- 1 3/4 tsp Lakanto monk fruit brilliant can utilize pretty much to change the sweetness
- 1/4 tsp preparing powder
- pinch of salt
- 1 tbsp Lily's Chocolate Chips

Directions

5. Turn on the waffle creator with the goal that it warms up.

6. In a little bowl, join all ingredients with the exception of the chocolate chips and mix well until consolidated.

7. Grease waffle producer, at that point, pour half of the hitter onto the base plate of the waffle creator.

8. Cook it for 5 minutes or until the chocolate chip chaffle pastry is brilliant dark colored at that point expel from waffle creator with a fork, being mindful so as not to burn your fingers.

Keto Strawberry Cheesecake Shake

Ingredients

- 1 cup Almond Milk, unsweetened
- 2oz Cream cheddar
- 1/2 cup Strawberries
- 2 tbsp Heavy cream
- 1 tbsp Lakanto monk fruit, or decision of sugar
- 1/2 tsp Vanilla
- 1 tbsp ChocZero Strawberry Syrup, discretionary

Directions

2. Add every one of the ingredients into a blender and mix until smooth. Include ice-blocks varying. Appreciate!

Keto Taco Chaffle Recipe (Crispy Taco Shells)

Ingredients

- 1 egg white

- 1/4 cup Monterey jack cheddar, destroyed (stuffed firmly)
- 1/4 cup sharp cheddar, destroyed (stuffed firmly)
- 3/4 tsp water
- 1 tsp coconut flour
- 1/4 tsp preparing powder
- 1/8 tsp stew powder
- pinch of salt

Directions

4. Plug the Dash Mini Waffle Maker in the divider and oil delicately once it is hot.

5. Combine the entirety of the ingredients in a bowl and mix to consolidate.

6. Spoon out 1/2 of the player on the waffle creator and close top. Set a clock for 4 minutes and don't lift the cover until the cooking time is finished. In the event that you do, it will resemble the taco chaffle shell isn't set up appropriately. However it will. You need to let it cook the whole 4 minutes before lifting the cover.

Maple Pumpkin Keto Waffle Recipe (Chaffle)

Ingredients

- 2 eggs
- 3/4 tsp heating powder
- 2 tsp pumpkin puree (100% pumpkin)
- 3/4 tsp pumpkin pie zest

- 4 tsp substantial whipping cream
- 2 tsp Lakanto Sugar-Free Maple Syrup
- 1 tsp coconut flour
- 1/2 cup mozzarella cheddar, destroyed
- 1/2 tsp vanilla
- pinch of salt

Guidelines

6. Turn on a waffle or chaffle producer. I utilize the Dash Mini Waffle Maker.
7. In a little bowl, join all ingredients.
8. Cover the scramble mini waffle producer with 1/4 of the player and cook for 3-4 minutes.
9. Repeat 3 additional occasions until you have made 4 Maple Syrup Pumpkin Keto Waffles (Chaffles).
10. Serve with without sugar maple syrup or keto frozen yogurt.

Keto Chaffle Breakfast Sandwich

Ingredients

- 1 egg
- 1/2 cup Monterey Jack Cheese
- 1 tablespoon almond flour
- 2 tablespoons spread

Directions

5. In a little bowl, blend the egg, almond flour, and Monterey Jack Cheese.

6. Pour a portion of the hitter into your mini waffle creator and cook for 3-4 minutes. At that point, cook the remainder of the player to make a second chaffle.

7. In a little container, dissolve 2 tablespoons of spread. Include the chaffles and cook each side for 2 minutes. Pushing down while they are cooking gently on the highest point of them, so they are fresh up better.

8. Remove from the container and let sit for 2 minutes.

Mini Keto Pizza Recipe

Ingredients

- 1/2 cup Shredded Mozzarella cheddar
- 1 tablespoon almond flour
- 1/2 tsp heating powder
- 1 egg
- 1/4 tsp garlic powder
- 1/4 tsp basil
- 2 tablespoons low carb pasta sauce
- 2 tablespoons mozzarella cheddar

Guidelines

4. While the waffle producer is warming up, in a bowl blend mozzarella cheddar, preparing powder, garlic, premise, egg, and almond flour.

5. Pour 1/2 the blend into your mini waffle producer.

6. Cook it for 3-5 min. until your pizza waffle is totally cooked. On the off chance that you check it and the waffle adheres to the waffle creator, let it cook for one more moment or two.

Sugar-Free Vanilla Buttercream Frosting

Ingredients

- 1 cup margarine room temperature
- 1.5 cups swerve confectioner
- 2 tbsp Heavy Whipping Cream
- 1 tsp vanilla concentrate

Guidelines

4. Place your margarine and swerve in the bowl of your blender. Combine them on low speed until the sugar is joined.

5. Mix in the substantial cream and the vanilla concentrate.

6. Turn the blender up to medium-fast and keep blending for 6-8 minutes until light and feathery.

Keto Blueberry Chaffle

This scrumptious keto blueberry waffles are, in fact, called a Keto Chaffle! What's more, a kid is it delish! Consummately sweet, with succulent blueberries, these blueberry keto chaffles taste extraordinary and are low carb and keto well disposed.

Ingredients

- 1 cup of mozzarella cheddar
- 2 tablespoons almond flour
- 1 tsp preparing powder
- 2 eggs
- 1 tsp cinnamon
- 2 tsp of Swerve
- 3 tablespoon blueberries

Directions

5. Heat up your Dash mini waffle creator.
6. In a blending bowl include the mozzarella cheddar, almond flour, preparing powder, eggs, cinnamon, swerve, and blueberries. Blend well, so every one of the ingredients is combined.
7. Spray your mini waffle creator with non-stick cooking splash.
8. Add shortly less than 1/4 a cup of blueberry keto waffle hitter.

Bacon Cheddar Chaffles Recipe

- 1 egg
- 1.2 cup cheddar
- Bacon bits to taste
- Mix and cook until fresh.

Bacon Jalapeno Chaffles Recipe

6. 1/2 cup destroyed swiss/gruyere mix

7. 1 egg

8. 2 tablespoons cooked bacon pieces

9. 1 tablespoon diced crisp jalapenos

10. Cook until fresh. Works incredibly as a bun to a cheeseburger.

Keto Cauliflower Chaffles Recipe

You can make the most delightful keto cauliflower chaffle formula with only a bunch of ingredients and a couple of moments! This formula will be your new top choice!

Ingredients

- 1 cup riced cauliflower
- 1/4 Tbsp. Garlic Powder
- 1/4 Tbsp. Ground Black Pepper
- 1/2 Tbsp. Italian Seasoning
- 1/4 Tbsp. salt
- 1/2 cup destroyed mozzarella cheddar or destroyed Mexican mix cheddar
- 1 Egg
- 1/2 cup destroyed parmesan cheddar

Sandwich Bread Chaffles Recipe

- 1 egg

- 2 tablespoon almond flour
- 1 tablespoon mayo
- 1/8 Tbsp. heating powder
- 1 Tbsp. water
- Sweetener and garlic powder (discretionary)
- Makes 2 chaffles, and you can undoubtedly slice them down the middle for a bun.

Sweet Chaffles Recipes

To make chaffles sweet, the conceivable outcomes are inestimable! You can just utilize the base formula and include some Keto-accommodating sugars.

In the event that you need to include some sweet seasoning after, you can sprinkle a wide range of Keto-accommodating magnificence on top. I like to utilize this Lakanto Maple Syrup. Something else, on the off chance that you need more than that, you can use the recipes beneath!

Chocolate Brownie Chaffles

- Making the Keto Chocolate Brownies Batter.
- Stir and pour in the mini waffle producer.
- You can see the entire formula and a video here for how to make chocolate chaffles
- Cook 5-7 minutes until firm. – TwoSleevers

Mint Chocolate Broffle (Brownie Waffle)

- Use this keto brownie formula.
- Add hacked walnuts, and each broffle (brownie waffle) utilized 3 tablespoons of player for 7 min.
- The formula for the buttercream depends on Urvashi's maple walnut buttercream formula, just with mint rather than maple separate.

Lemon Pound Cake Chaffles

Numerous individuals are cutting my lemon pound cake formula by 1/4 and making Cake Chaffles out of them.

Crusty fruit-filled treat CHAFFLES

- 1.2 cup mozzarella cheddar
- 1 egg
- Add the mozzarella to the waffle producer.
- Put the egg on top.
- Sprinkle on crusty fruit-filled treat zest and 5 sugar-free chocolate chips.
- Serve with margarine on top.

Cream Cheese Carrot Cake Chaffles

- 2 tablespoons cream cheddar or a blend of 1 tablespoon cream cheddar and 2 tablespoons destroyed mozzarella cheddar
- 1/2 pat of margarine
- 1 tablespoon finely destroyed carrot

- 1 tablespoon of sugar of your decision. I utilized Splenda.
- 1 tablespoon almond flour
- 1 Tbsp. pumpkin pie zest
- 1/2 Tbsp. vanilla
- 1/2 Tbsp. heating powder
- 1 egg

Optional

I included 6 raisins, 1 tablespoon of destroyed coconut, and 1/2 tablespoon of pecans to the blender ingredients.

Cream Cheese Frosting

- 1 tablespoon cream cheddar
- 1 pat spread
- 1 Tbsp. sugar of decision. I utilized Cinnamon Brown Sugar without sugar syrup.
- Heat up, waffle creator. I utilized a mini Dash. I oiled with a silicon brush dunked in coconut oil.
- Microwave cream cheddar, mozzarella, and spread for 15 seconds to liquefy the cheeses to make consolidating simpler. I did this in an enchantment slug cup to mix.
- Add the remainder of the chaffle ingredients to the blender cup and mix until smooth and consolidated.
- Add a player to a waffle creator. For the Dash, I included 2 stacking tablespoons, and it made 3 chaffles.

- While making the chaffle, heat up the spread and cream cheddar for the icing. Blend until smooth, and consolidate your sugar. Sprinkle over chaffles as wanted.

Cinnamon Chaffles

- 1/2 cup mozzarella
- 1 egg
- 1 tbsp vanilla concentrate
- 1/2 tsp preparing powder
- 1 tbsp almond flour
- Sprinkle of cinnamon
- Mix together and cook until chaffles are firm.

Cinnamon Swirl Chaffles

- CHAFFLE:
- 1 oz cream cheddar, mollified
- 1 huge egg, beaten
- 1 tsp vanilla concentrate
- 1 tbsp almond flour, superfine
- 1 tbsp Splenda
- 1 tsp cinnamon
- ICING:
- 1 oz cream cheddar, mollified
- 1 tbsp. spread, unsalted

- 1 tbsp Splenda
- 1/2 tsp vanilla

Cinnamon Drizzle:

- 1/2 tbsp spread
- 1 tbsp Splenda
- 1 tsp cinnamon
- Heat up waffle creator, and I brushed on coconut oil on my DASH.
- Stir up the chaffle ingredients until smooth.
- Utilize a spoon to include 2 piling tbsp of the player to the waffle iron. It will make 3 little waffles.
- Cook to your ideal waffle freshness. I did 4 min. They resembled a delicate waffle.
- Cool on a rack.
- Mix the icing and cinnamon shower in little dishes. Warmth in the microwave for 10 secs to find a workable pace consistency. Whirl on cooled waffles.

Greek Marinated Feta And Olives

Ingredients

- 1 cup olive oil
- 1/4 Tbsp. oregano
- 1/4 Tbsp. thyme
- 1/2 Tbsp. dried rosemary
- 1 cup kalamata olives

- 1 cup of green olives
- 1/2 pound feta

Directions

- In a little pot heat, the oil, oregano, thyme, rosemary together over medium warmth for 5 minutes to imbue the oil with the herbs.
- Set the oil to the side and enable it to cool for 15 minutes.
- Cut the feta into 1/2 inch 3D shapes.

Air Fryer Peanut Chicken

Not many things state "Thai food" like Peanut Chicken. This Peanut Chicken formula takes the dish to an unheard-of level and is effectively made in your air fryer!

Ingredients

- 1 pound Bone-in Skin-on Chicken Thighs
- For the Sauce
- 1/4 cup Creamy Peanut Butter
- 1 tablespoon Sriracha Sauce, (modify for your zest needs)
- 1 tablespoon Soy Sauce
- 2 tablespoons sweet chili sauce
- 2 tablespoons lime juice
- 1 Tbsp. Minced Garlic
- 1 Tbsp. minced ginger
- 1/2 Tbsp. salt, to taste
- 1/2 cup high temp water

Green Beans With Bacon

Right now, Pot Green Beans with Bacon formula is a fast, low carb, and nutritious dish that can be eaten either as a side dish or as a low carb dinner. Just beans, bacon, and a couple of seasonings make this a quick and simple dish.

Ingredients

- 1 cup (160 g) onion, diced
- 5 cuts (5 cuts) Bacon, diced
- 6 cups (660 g) green beans, cut in

Keto Buffalo Chicken Casserole

This Buffalo Chicken Casserole is as flavorful filling dish with the perfect measure of kick! It's the ideal weeknight supper that requires little exertion to make.

Ingredients

- 4 cups rotisserie chicken, destroyed
- 1/2 cup Onion, slashed
- 1/4 cup Cream
- 1/4 cup hot wing sauce
- 1/4 cup blue cheddar, disintegrated
- 2 ounces Cream Cheese, diced
- pepper
- 1/4 cup Green Onions, slashed

German Red Cabbage

Appreciate this customary German Red Cabbage formula made in a non-conventional way! Make this wonderfully prepared side dish directly in your Instant Pot!

Ingredients

- 6 cups red cabbage, cleaved
- 3 Granny Smith Apples, little, cut 1 inch thick
- 2 tablespoons liquefied margarine, or oil
- 1/3 cup Apple Cider Vinegar
- 2-3 tablespoons Sugar
- 1 Tbsp. salt
- 1/2 Tbsp. Ground Black Pepper
- 1/4 Tbsp. Ground Cloves
- 2 sound leaves

Maple Pecan Bars With Sea Salt

Ingredients

For the Crust

- Non-Stick Spray
- 1/3 cup Butter, mellowed
- 1/4 cup Brown Sugar, immovably stuffed
- 1 cup All-Purpose Flour
- 1/4 Kosher tea Salt

For the Filling

- 4 TBS Butter (1/2 stick), diced
- 1/2 cup Brown Sugar
- 1/4 cup Pure Maple Syrup
- 1/4 cup Whole Milk
- 1/4 tea Vanilla concentrate

Moment Pot Vegetarian Chili

Ingredients

- 1 cup Onion, cleaved
- 1 cup Canned Fire Roasted Tomatoes
- 1.5 tablespoons Minced Garlic
- 3 corn tortillas
- 1 tablespoon Chipotle Chile in Adobo Sauce, cleaved
- 1 tablespoon Mexican Red Chili Powder, (not cayenne)
- 2 Tbsp.s Ground Cumin
- 2 Tbsp.s salt
- 1 Tbsp. Dried Oregano
- 1 cup Water
- 1/2 cup dried pinto beans, doused medium-term or for 1 hour in heated water
- 1/2 cup dried dark beans, splashed medium-term or for 1 hour in high temp water
- 2 cups corn, new or defrosted solidified corn

- 2 cups zucchini, hacked

Keto Almendrados Cookies | Spanish Almond Keto Cookies

Ingredients

- 1.5 cups Superfine Almond Flour
- 1/2 cup Swerve
- 1 huge Egg
- 1 Tbsp. Lemon Extract
- 1 tablespoon lemon get-up-and-go
- 24 whitened almonds

Directions

4. In a medium bowl, beat egg. Include almond flour, swerve and lemon and combine to make a strong mixture. Cover and refrigerate for 1-2 hours.

5. Preheat stove to 350 degrees. Line a heating sheet with material paper.

6. Pinching off bits of batter about the size of a pecan, fold them into balls.

Keto Taco

Prep. time: 11 minutes/Cook time: 20 minutes/Serves 3

Need to begin the day surprising? Morning keto is such an astounding beginning to a delightful day. Light and superb with a lot of splendid hues and feelings.

8 oz. Mozzarella cheddar, destroyed; 6 Eggs, enormous 2 tbsp. Margarine

3 Bacon stripes ½ Avocado 1 oz. Cheddar, destroyed Pepper and salt to taste

Keto Omelet With Goat Cheese And Spinach

Prep. time: 5 minutes

3 Large eggs 1 Medium green onion 1 oz. Goat cheddar ¼ Onion

2 tbsp. Margarine 2 cups Spinach 2 tbsp. Substantial cream Salt and pepper to taste

Chicken And Cheese Quesadilla

Prep. time: 10 minutes/Serves 4

For capsules: 6 Eggs 4 oz. Coconut flour 6 oz. Substantial cream ½ tsp. Thickener Pink salt and pepper 1 tbsp. Olive oil for fricasseeing

For the quesadilla: 4 oz. Cheddar destroyed 8 oz. Chicken bosom cooked and destroyed 1 tbsp. Parsley, cleaved (discretionary)

Gluten Free Sports Nutrition Basics

At the point when you're a competitor, it's imperative to get a decent assortment of protein, sugars, and sound fats for the duration of the day. Evading gluten implies picking gluten-free nourishments and wiping out wheat, grain, and rye items from your eating routine to keep away from aggravation, swelling, stomach torment, cramps, looseness of the bowels, exhaustion, lack of healthy sustenance, iron deficiency, and blockage.

Protein Needs

The American College of Sports Medicine and the Academy of Nutrition and Dietetics prescribe athletes eat 0.5 to 0.8 grams of protein per pound of their body weight day by day, and 15 to 20 percent of their complete calories from protein.

Pick a lot of protein-rich nourishments, for example,

- Lean meats, poultry, fish, and fish
- Eggs
- Low-fat dairy nourishments or dairy substitutes
- Tofu or other soy items
- Legumes
- Nuts, seeds, and nut margarines

Carb Requirements

Carbs are essential for athletes since this macronutrient is a competitor's primary vitality source. Athletes get 50 to 60 percent of their calories from carbs, or 2.7 to 4.6 grams of carbs per pound of body weight day by day. Pick sound, gluten-free carbs, for example,

- Gluten-free oats, oats, and oats (must indicate gluten-free)
- Rice
- Quinoa
- Fruits
- Starchy vegetables like potatoes, yams, peas, corn, and vegetables

Fat Recommendations

Dietary fat should make up around 20 to 30 percent of a competitor's calorie consumption. Pick sound fats, for example,

- Nuts and seeds
- Nut margarines
- Plant-based oils
- Avocadoes
- Olives

Gluten Free Recipes for Athletes

Gluten Free Recipes For Athletes

The accompanying gluten-free recipes make certain to be a hit with athletes, regardless of whether utilized before working out for a snappy increase in vitality or as a post-practice recuperation feast or bite.

Almond Blast Protein Shake

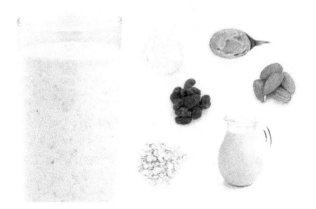

This shake assists athletes with devouring protein, which is basic for muscle improvement.

Fixings

- 2 scoops of gluten-free vanilla-seasoned protein powder
- 1.5 cups of low-fat milk, soy milk, or almond milk
- ½ cup of gluten-free oats
- ½ cup of raisins
- 12 fragmented almonds
- 1 tablespoon of nutty spread

Bearings

Mix all fixings together in blender and serve chilled.

Chocolate Peanut Butter Protein Balls

Anoth er protein-rich formula, these protein balls make an incredible pre- or post-exercise nibble.

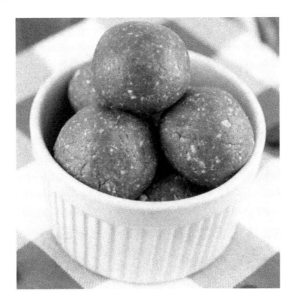

Fixings

- 1 cup of gluten-free moved oats
- 1/2 cup of characteristic nutty spread
- 1/3 cup of nectar
- 2 tablespoons of flax seeds
- 2 tablespoons of chia seeds
- 1 tablespoon of gluten-free chocolate protein powder

Bearings

5.   Stir all fixings together in a bowl.

6.   Cover the bowl with cling wrap.

7.   Refrigerate blend for 30 minutes.

8.   Scoop chilled blend into balls and serve.

Tomato Spinach Omelet

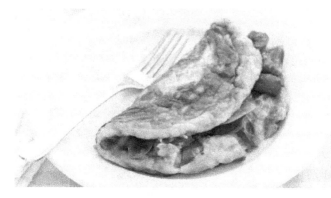

With sound protein and nutrient-thick veggies, this formula is an extraordinary method to begin the day.

Fixings

- 4 enormous eggs
- 1/2 cup broiler cooked tomatoes
- 1 cup infant spinach leaves
- 1/2 cup feta cheddar
- 1 tablespoon olive oil

Headings

8. Saute the spinach and tomatoes in the olive oil over medium-low warmth for a few minutes.

9. Pour the beaten eggs into the skillet and gradually shake to circulate equitably all through.

10. After around two minutes, slacken the omelet blend from the base of the container to forestall staying.

11. Sprinkle the feta cheddar over the omelet.

12. Fold the omelet with the cheddar in the center and cook until it is brilliant darker.

13. Flip the omelet and cook for one increasingly minute.

14. Serve with gluten-free toast and orange cuts, whenever wanted.

Quinoa And Asparagus Chicken Salad

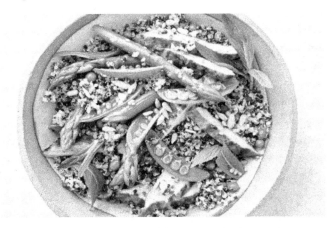

This formula is an extraordinary wellspring of gluten-free complex carbs and protein.

Fixings

- 1/2 cup uncooked quinoa

- 2 ounces chicken bosom
- 1/2 cup sun-dried tomatoes
- 10-ounces asparagus
- 1/2 cup feta cheddar
- 1 tablespoon olive oil
- Salt and pepper

Headings

6. Cook the quinoa as guided and add it to an enormous bowl.

7. Steam the asparagus for around 5 minutes and cut it into little pieces.

8. Add the asparagus, tomatoes, feta cheddar, and chicken bosom to bowl with the quinoa.

9. Add the olive oil, salt, and pepper.

10. Mix all fixings and appreciate!

Turkey Chili

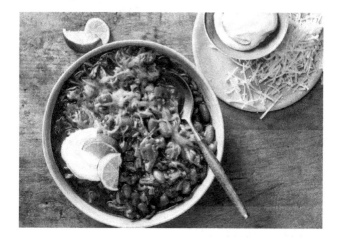

Lean protein, complex carbs, and bunches of flavor makes this a thought formula for athletes.

Fixings

- 2 cups water
- 1 pound ground turkey
- 1 jar of diced tomatoes
- 1 jar of kidney beans
- 1 slashed onion
- 1 1/2 Tbsp.s olive oil
- 1 tablespoon minced garlic
- 2 tablespoons bean stew powder
- 1/2 Tbsp. oregano
- 1/2 Tbsp. ground cumin
- 1/2 Tbsp. paprika
- Salt and pepper to taste

Headings

5. Cook the turkey and olive oil in a pot over medium warmth until darker.
6. Add the onions and cook until delicate.
7. Add the rest of the fixings and heat the blend to the point of boiling.
8. Reduce the warmth to low and stew for about 30 minutes.

Anti-Aging Recipes

Edamame With Ground Bonito And Seaweed

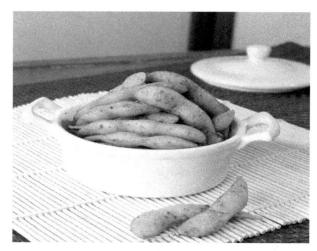

Prep Time: 5 Minutes/ Cook Time: 6 Minutes/ Total Time: 11 Minutes/

Category: Snack/ Cuisine: Vegetarian

Fixings

- 1 pound edamame (new or solidified)
- 1/4 nori sheet
- 2 tablespoons bonito chips
- 1/2 Tbsp. salt

Directions

4. Follow bearings on edamame bundle on how to cook them (I lean toward bubbling them two or three minutes not as much as

what the headings state, as it makes them less soft). Channel them and let them dry for 2-3 minutes.

5. Break the nori and add it to an espresso/flavor processor alongside the bonito pieces and the salt. Granulate the blend until it nearly transforms into a powder.

6. Put the edamame in a blending bowl and sprinkle the powdered blend over them. Hurl a couple of times and serve.

Korean Pickles

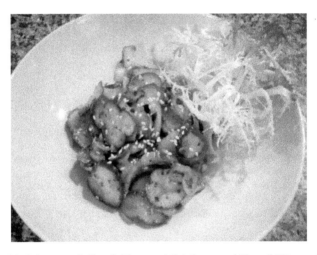

Prep Time: 10 Minutes/ Cook Time: 15 Minutes/ Total Time: 25 Minutes/ Category: Condiment/ Cuisine: Korean

Fixings

- 2 cups daikon (stripped and julienned (cut into little strips))
- 1 medium carrot (stripped and julienned)
- 1 shallot (finely hacked)

- 2 tablespoons water

- 3 tablespoons rice vinegar

- 2 Tbsp.s tobanjan (Korean stew glue)

- 2 Tbsp.s sesame oil

- 1 Tbsp. granulated sugar

- 2 Tbsp.s salt (in addition to included 1/2 Tbsp.)

- 1 tablespoon sesame seeds

Directions

5. Put the daikon, carrots and shallot in a medium size blending bowl and include 2 tsp salt. Rapidly blend in with your hands and leave for 10 minutes, to mollify the veggies.

6. In a different little bowl, blend water, rice vinegar and tobanjan. Mix until tobanjan has weakened and include sugar, 1/2 tsp salt, and sesame oil. Mix well until sugar and salt have dissolved.

7. Rinse the vegetable, channel and press out overabundance water. Return the vegetable in the blending bowl and pour the tobanjan blend over.

8. Add sesame seeds and utilizing chopsticks or a spoon, blend until veggies are all around covered. Serve or let pickle for as long as 3 days.

Nourishment

- Calories: 233

- Saturated Fat: 2

Pan Fried Food Beef With Spicy Hoisin Sauce

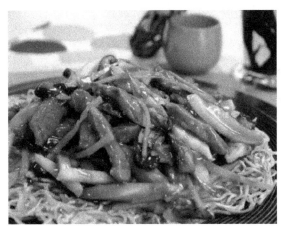

Make this hot, valid Szechuan hoisin pan sear hamburger formula in under 20 minutes!

Prep Time: 10 Minutes/ Cook Time: 6 Minutes/ Total Time: 16 Minutes/ Yield: 2 People 1x/ Category: Main/ Cuisine: Chinese

Fixings

- 1/2 pound lean meat (meagerly cut scaled down)
- 1 red chime pepper (center and seeded, cut into meager strips (julienne))
- 4 scallions (generally cleaved)
- 1 tablespoon vegetable oil
- 2 cloves garlic (finely cleaved)
- 2 Thai bean stews (finely slashed)
- 2 tablespoons hoisin sauce
- 1 Tbsp. white miso glue

- For the marinade:
- 1 tablespoon dull soy
- 1 tablespoon soy sauce
- 1 tablespoon shaoxing wine or dry sherry
- 1 tablespoon corn starch

Directions

6. Put all the element for the marinade in a bowl with the meat. Blend well and put in a safe spot for 30 minutes.

7. In a medium size container over high warmth, include oil, garlic and chiles and cook for 1 moment.

8. Add meat and cook for 3 minutes.

9. Add pepper and scallions and cook for 2 minutes, mixing regularly.

10. Turn the warmth off, include hoisin sauce and miso glue, mix well until glue has broken up. Serve pan sear with white rice.

Notes

This Stir Fry Beef With Hoisin Sauce:

Exceptionally high in iron

High in selenium

Extremely high in nutrient B6

Extremely high in nutrient B12

Extremely high in nutrient C

High in zinc

Sauteed Kale With Mustard Sauce

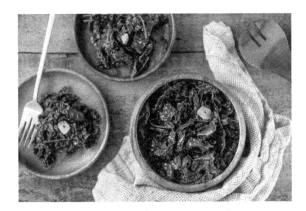

Prep Time: 5 Minutes/ Cook Time: 7 Minutes/ Total Time: 12 Minutes/

Yield: 2 1x/ Category: Side

Fixings

- 2 tablespoons additional virgin olive oil
- 1 clove garlic (minced)
- 1/4 cup white wine
- 1 pack kale (ribs expelled and finely hacked)
- 1/2 Tbsp. genuine salt
- 1/4 Tbsp. ground dark pepper
- 1 Tbsp. dijon mustard
- 1/4 cup milk

Directions

6. In a container over medium/high warmth, include olive oil and garlic. Cook for 1 moment.

7. Add white wine, mix well and cook for 1 moment.

8. Add kale, mix well and cook for 4 minutes, mixing continually.

9. Add salt and pepper, mix and cook for 1 moment.

10. Turn off the warmth, include milk and dijon mustard and rapidly mix until fluid is no more. Serve.

Sauteed Green Beans With Chilies

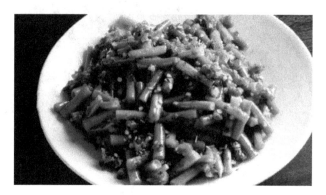

Prep Time: 10 Minutes/ Cook Time: 5 Minutes/ Total Time: 15 Minutes/ Yield: 4 1x/ Category: Side/ Cuisine: Chinese

Fixings

- 2 cloves garlic (finely hacked)
- 1 Tbsp. ginger (stripped and finely hacked)
- 1 pound green beans (washed)
- 2 tablespoons vegetable oil
- 1 Tbsp. dried red chilies (hacked)
- 1 tablespoon shellfish sauce
- 1 tablespoon soy sauce
- 1 Tbsp. sesame oil

Directions

7. Bring a pot of salted water to bubble (not as salty as the ocean, yet enough that you can taste it).

8. Meanwhile, flush and cut the parts of the bargains bean.

9. When water is bubbling, whiten the green beans for 3 minutes. Channel.

10. In a medium size container, include the vegetable oil, garlic, ginger and dried chilies. Cook for a moment and include green beans.

11. Toss and cook for one more moment, at that point include soy sauce and clam sauce.

12. Toss well, include sesame oil and turn the warmth off. Serve.

Nourishment

- Calories: 109
- Saturated Fat: 1

Shrimp And Celery Salad With Wasabi Mayo

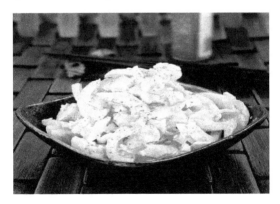

Prep Time: 10 Minutes/ Cook Time: 5 Minutes/ Total Time: 15 Minutes/
Yield: 4 Sides 1x/ Category: Salads/ Method: Chopping/ Cuisine:
Japanese

Fixings

- 16–20 huge crude shrimps, deveined and stripped
- 3 celery stalks, cleaved reduced down
- 2 tablespoon orange, red or green chime peppers, diced
- 1/4 cup mayonnaise
- 1/2 tablespoon rice vinegar
- 1/2 Tbsp. wasabi glue
- Salt and ichimi togarashi to taste

Directions

7. Bring a little pot of water with 1 tablespoon salt to bubble.

8. Add celery and heat up (this procedure is called whitening) for 2 minutes. Channel and wash celery in cool water. Put in a safe spot.

9. Bring another little pot of water to bubble, include shrimps and bubble for 3 minutes. Channel, wash in chilly water and put in a safe spot.

10. In a medium size blending bowl, mix mayonnaise, rice vinegar and wasabi glue together until smooth.

11. Dry the shrimps with a paper towel or hand towel, and slash them into reduced down. Add to the blending bowl.

12. Add celery and ringer peppers to the blending bowl, and mix the entirety of the fixings well. Season with salt and pepper. Serve cold.

Notes

This shrimp and celery serving of mixed greens will keep refrigerated in a hermetically sealed compartment for as long as 2 days.

Fish Steak With Tomato Relish

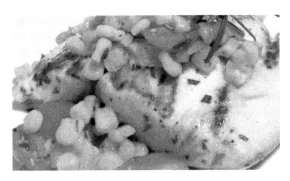

Prep Time: 5 Minutes/ Cook Time: 17 Minutes/ Total Time: 22 Minutes/ Yield: 2 1x/ Category: Main/ Cuisine: Fish, Seafood

Fixings

- 2 pounds fish steak
- 3 tablespoons additional virgin olive oil
- 1 clove garlic (finely hacked)
- 1 half quart treasure or cherry tomatoes (finely hacked)
- 1/2 medium onion (finely hacked)
- 8 leaves new basil (generally hacked)
- 1 Tbsp. sugar

- salt and pepper to taste
- lemon wedges (to serve)

Directions

3. In a dish over high warmth, include 2 tbsp olive oil, garlic and onions, and cook for 3-4 minutes, until onions are translucent. Include tomatoes and sugar, and cook for 5 minutes, or until the blend is practically similar to a sauce. Mood killer the warmth, include basil and season with salt, and pepper.

4. Use a different dish to cook the fish. Season the fish with salt and pepper on the two sides. Hold up until the dish is hot and include the staying 1 tbsp olive oil. Include fish steaks and lower the warmth to medium/high. Spread and cook until all around done (around 7 minutes). Covering the dish keeps the fish clammy, I utilize this stunt for fish, chicken and even meat; it has exactly the intended effect.

Nourishment

- Calories: 655
- Saturated Fat: 4

Stout Vegetable Soup

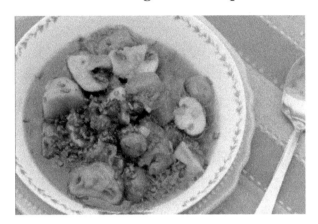

Prep Time: 15 Minutes/ Cook Time: an hour/ Total Time: 75 Minutes/ Yield: 4 People 1x/ Category: Soup/ Cuisine: Vegetarian/ Scale 1x2x3x

Fixings

- 3 cloves garlic (finely hacked)
- 1 onion (finely hacked)
- 3 tablespoons additional virgin olive oil
- 3 medium carrots (generally cleaved)
- 2 stalks celery (generally cleaved)
- 2 turnips (generally cleaved)
- 1/4 head cabbage (generally cleaved)
- 28 oz can squashed tomatoes
- 7 cups vegetable stock
- 1/2 Tbsp. dried thyme
- dried herbs like basil oregano as well as parsley

- salt and pepper (to taste)

Directions

4. In a huge pot over high warmth, include oil, garlic, dried thyme and onions. Cook for 4-6 minutes until onions relax and turn out to be clear. Include the squashed tomatoes and mix. Include everything else; carrots, celery, turnips, cabbage, vegetable juices and dried herbs. Season with somewhat salt and bring to bubble.

5. Bring to bubble, spread and lower warmth to a stew. Cook for 25 minutes or until vegetables are cooked through. Keep an eye on your soup on occasion and mix to ensure veggies aren't consuming at the base of the pot.

6. Season with salt and pepper and serve.

Notes

This stout vegetable soup can likewise be presented with new cleaved parsley and wafers.

CPSIA information can be obtained
at www.ICGtesting.com
Printed in the USA
LVHW101143191120
672145LV00012B/403